Pharmaceutical Calculations

The Pharmacist's Handbook

Pharmaceutical Calculations

The Pharmacist's Handbook

Howard C. Ansel, PhD
Professor and Dean Emeritus
College of Pharmacy
The University of Georgia
Athens, Georgia

Shelly J. Prince, RPh, PhD
Associate Professor of Pharmaceutics
Department of Pharmaceutical Sciences
School of Pharmacy
Southwestern Oklahoma State University
Weatherford, Oklahoma

LIPPINCOTT WILLIAMS & WILKINS
A Wolters Kluwer Company
Philadelphia • Baltimore • New York • London
Buenos Aires • Hong Kong • Sydney • Tokyo

Editor: David B. Troy
Managing Editor: Matthew J. Hauber
Marketing Manager: Chris Kushner
Production Editor: Jennifer D. Weir
Designer: Doug Smock
Compositor: Maryland Composition
Printer: RR Donnelley

351 West Camden Street
Baltimore, MD 21201

530 Walnut Street
Philadelphia, PA 19106

Printed in the United States of America

Library of Congress Cataloging-in-Publication Data

Ansel, Howard C., 1933-
Pharmaceutical calculations: the pharmacist's handbook / Howard C. Ansel, Shelly J. Prince.
p. cm.
Includes index.
ISBN 0-7817-3922-5
1. Pharmaceutical arithmetic. I. Prince, Shelly J. II. Title.

RS57.A57 2003
615'.1'015—dc21

2003047625

03 04 05 06 07
1 2 3 4 5 6 7 8 9 10

PREFACE

This, the first edition of *Pharmaceutical Calculations: The Pharmacist's Handbook*, provides a ready reference to pharmaceutical calculations directly applicable to the practice of pharmacy.

The *Handbook* is designed for pharmacy students who have an understanding of the fundamentals of pharmaceutical calculations and are engaged in practice laboratories or in the internship/externship/clerkship components of the professional curriculum. The *Handbook* is also a resource for pharmacy graduates preparing for licensure examinations, for pharmacists in everyday practice, and for those serving as preceptors or part-time faculty.

Based on the more definitive work, *Pharmaceutical Calculations*, 11th edition, by Howard C. Ansel and Mitchell J. Stoklosa, the *Handbook* contains the broad array of calculations essential to the practice of pharmacy in a format designed for ease of use as a reference and resource. This is accomplished through the *Handbook's* physical size; design features; organizational system of parts, chapters, and sections; and uniform format of topical headings and content. The *Handbook's* 20 chapters are organized by general subject matter and presented in logical sequence. This permits a systematic approach for both a start-to-finish use of the *Handbook*, as well as the location of a specific type of calculation. A final part, "Competency Assessment," permits self-assessment through an exercise of comprehensive and integrated practice problems. Appendices include resource information pertinent to various types of calculations. Compared with the primary text, the *Handbook* is more concise in its explanations and problem sets and contains added subject matter befitting the academic level and needs of advanced students and practitioners.

Acknowledgments

The authors are grateful to faculty and student reviewers of this work, who gave thoughtful impressions of the conceptual idea for the *Handbook* and later offered their specific and helpful comments on the prepared manuscript.

Acknowledgment is made to Daniel Limmer, who conceived of the idea for the *Handbook*, and to Lippincott Williams & Wilkins associates Matt Hauber, David Troy, and others, whose support and expertise were drawn on throughout the process. Special gratitude is expressed to Barry Gales and ElGenia French for their valuable input and to Mitchell J. Stoklosa for his generosity in allowing liberal use of the text *Pharmaceutical Calculations* in the preparation of this work.

Howard C. Ansel
Athens, Georgia

Shelly J. Prince
Weatherford, Oklahoma

TABLE OF CONTENTS

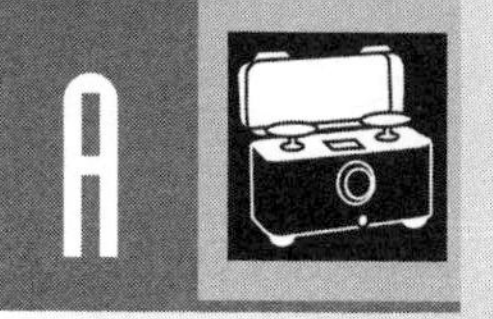

Fundamental Systems and Methods of Pharmaceutical Calculations

1

BASIC METHODS

This chapter presents two common methods for use in solving many of the pharmaceutical calculations problems presented in this *Handbook* and encountered in pharmacy practice. They are: ratio and proportion, and dimensional analysis. Preference for either of these methods generally is based on a pharmacist's experience and comfort with the particular method. Dimensional analysis is the method most used in this *Handbook*. For further explanation of either of these methods, the reader is directed to the references at the end of this chapter.[1,2]

1.1 Ratio and Proportion

Many of the calculations problems that pharmacists encounter may be solved through the use of properly set up ratios and proportions.

Definitions. The relative magnitude of two like quantities is called their ratio (e.g., 1:4). A proportion is the expression of the equality of two ratios (e.g., 1:4 = 4:16).

Expression. A ratio, describing the relative magnitude of its two numbers, may be expressed as a common fraction (e.g., 1/4) or more traditionally by the use of colons (e.g., 1:4). However, with either manner of presentation,

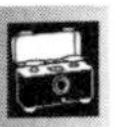

the ratio is not read as a fraction, that is, not as "one-fourth" but as "1 to 4." A ratio may be of abstract numbers, or it may be associated with units.

For example:

The ratio 1:1,000 is expressed as "1 to 1,000," or "1 part to 1,000 parts,"
The ratio 2 g:500 g is expressed as "2 g to 500 g," and
The ratio 3 mL:25 mL is expressed as "3 mL to 25 mL."

In a ratio, the first term, or numerator, may be larger or smaller than the second term, or denominator (e.g., 5:1 or 1:5), with the value of the ratio determined by dividing the first term by the second term. The units of a ratio must be the same when its value is calculated to determine how many times greater or smaller the first term is than the second term. When two ratios have the same value, they are equivalent and are proportional one to the other. For example, the ratio 1:5 has a value of 0.2, as does the ratio 5:25, and thus they are equivalent and proportional.

A proportion may be written in any one of three standard forms:

(1) $a:b = c:d$ (e.g., $1:5 = 5:25$)
(2) $a:b :: c:d$ (e.g., $1:5 :: 5:25$)
(3) $\frac{a}{b} = \frac{c}{d} \left(\text{e.g., } \frac{1}{5} = \frac{5}{25}\right)$

Each of these expressions is read: a is to b as c is to d (or 1 is to 5 as 5 is to 25).

Discussion. The arithmetic rules governing common fractions equally apply to ratios. Thus, if both terms of a ratio (the numerator and denominator) are multiplied or are divided by the same number, the value remains

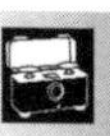

unchanged. For example, when both terms of the ratio 20:4 are multiplied by 2, yielding 40:8, or divided by 2, yielding 10:2, the quotient (the value of 5) remains the same. It is often useful to reduce the terms of a ratio by use of a common divisor. For example, the ratio 2:250 may be reduced by dividing both terms by 2, resulting in an equivalent ratio of 1:125.

An interesting fact about equivalent ratios is that the product of the numerator of one and the denominator of the other always equals the product of the denominator of the one and the numerator of the other; in other words, the cross-products are equal. Or, as is commonly stated, the product of the extremes equals the product of the means, the extremes being the "outer" numbers and the means being the "inner" numbers. This fact may be demonstrated with the following equivalent ratios, $\frac{2}{4} = \frac{4}{8}$ in which the product of the extremes (2×8) and the product of the means (4×4) each equal 16.

This is the basis for the use of ratio and proportion in many pharmaceutical calculations. In any proportion, when three of the terms are known, the fourth (or missing) term can easily be calculated.

Although not necessary, the traditional pattern for the setup of a proportion is to place the unknown term (designated x) in the second fraction. Then, solving for x yields the answer. For example:

$$\frac{5}{100} = \frac{x}{60};\ 100\ x = 300;\ x = \frac{300}{100};\ x = 3.$$

Key Point. A valid proportion is based on the equivalency of two ratios. When terms or units are associated with the quantities of one ratio, identical terms or units must be associated with the second ratio of the proportion. For example, if one ratio states that there are 5 g of

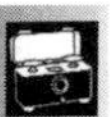

a component in 25 mL of a preparation, the second ratio of the proportion must also relate grams to milliliters. These are termed mixed ratios in a proportion, and invoke the principle that if the ratios are regarded as abstract numbers, the means or the extremes may be interchanged without destroying the validity of the equation. Thus, a valid proportion may be written as:

$$\frac{5\text{ g}}{25\text{ mL}} = \frac{15\text{ g}}{75\text{ mL}} \quad \text{or as} \quad \frac{5\text{ g}}{15\text{ g}} = \frac{25\text{ mL}}{75\text{ mL}}$$

$$\text{or as} \quad \frac{75\text{ mL}}{25\text{ mL}} = \frac{15\text{ g}}{5\text{ g}}$$

In each instance, the ratios are equivalent.

Pharmacy Applications. Single ratios are used in pharmacy as an expression of the relative amount of one item compared with a second, commonly the quantity of one component of a preparation compared with the quantity of the total preparation (e.g., 1 g to 1,000 g or 1:1,000). This is termed ratio strength, a topic discussed in Chapter 4.

Equivalent ratios, or proportions, are used in solving the types of problems presented in the following example problems.

EXAMPLE PROBLEMS

1. If three tablets contain 975 mg of aspirin, how many milligrams of aspirin would be contained in 12 tablets?

   [The proportion may be set up as follows and read as: 3 tablets are to 975 mg as 12 tablets are to x (or "how many") mg?]

$$\frac{3\text{ (tablets)}}{975\text{ (mg)}} = \frac{12\text{ (tablets)}}{x\text{ (mg)}}$$

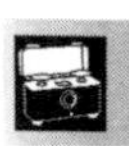

Then, solving arithmetically for x, we have:

$3x = 975 \times 12$, or

$x = \frac{975 \times 12}{3}$, and

$x = 3{,}900$ mg

2. If a cough syrup contains 2 mg of brompheniramine maleate in each 5-mL dose, how many milligrams of the agent would be contained in a 120-mL container of the syrup?

$$\frac{2\ (\text{mg})}{5\ (\text{mL})} = \frac{x\ (\text{mg})}{120\ (\text{mL})}$$

$$x = \frac{2 \times 120}{5}$$

$$x = 48\ \text{mg}$$

3. If a potassium chloride elixir contains 20 mEq of potassium ion in each 15 mL of elixir, how many milliliters will provide 25 mEq of potassium ion to the patient?

$$\frac{20\ (\text{mEq})}{15\ (\text{mL})} = \frac{25\ (\text{mEq})}{x\ (\text{mL})}$$

$$x = \frac{15 \times 25}{20}$$

$$x = 18.75\ \text{mL}$$

4. If a syringe contains 5 mg of medication in each 10 mL of solution, how many milligrams of medication would be administered when 4 mL of solution are injected?

$$\frac{5\ (\text{mg})}{10\ (\text{mL})} = \frac{x\ (\text{mg})}{4\ (\text{mL})}$$

$$x = \frac{5 \times 4}{10}$$

$$x = 2\ \text{mg}$$

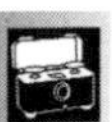

5. If a pediatric vitamin contains 1,500 units of vitamin A per milliliter of solution, how many units of vitamin A would be administered to a child given two drops of the solution from a dropper calibrated to deliver 20 drops per mL of solution?

$$\frac{20\ \text{(drops)}}{1\ \text{(mL)}} = \frac{2\ \text{(drops)}}{x\ \text{(mL)}}$$

$$x = \frac{2 \times 1}{20}$$

$x = 0.1$ mL, then

$$\frac{1\ \text{(mL)}}{1{,}500\ \text{(units)}} = \frac{0.1\ \text{(mL)}}{x\ \text{(units)}}$$

$$x = \frac{1{,}500 \times 0.1}{1}$$

$x = 150$ units

1.2 Dimensional Analysis

Definition. Dimensional analysis is a problem-solving method that applies needed equivalents and unit-conversion factors to ensure that the terms of an equation have the same dimensions.

Expression. The basic equation used in dimensional analysis is:

Given Quantities and Units × Equivalents and Unit-Conversion Factors = Answer in Desired Units

The equivalents and unit-conversion factors are selected to permit the cancellation of all undesired units in the equation while retaining the units desired in the answer. As shown in the example problems below, the numerators and denominators of the conversion factors must be correctly placed to allow the unwanted units to be canceled.

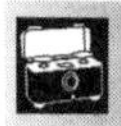

Discussion. When performing certain types of calculations, many pharmacists prefer to use dimensional analysis. By this method, ratios of the data are used, equivalents and unit-conversion factors are added as necessary, and some individual terms are inverted (to their reciprocals) to permit the cancellation of like units in the numerator(s) and denominators(s), leaving only the desired term(s) of the answer. An advantage to the use of dimensional analysis is the consolidation of multiple arithmetical steps into a single expression.

Key Point. In setting up an equation for solving by dimensional analysis, the units desired in the answer often are placed in the answer position before solving the arithmetic problem to guide the placement of the various terms of the equation, such that the undesired terms cancel out, leaving only terms desired in the answer.

Pharmacy Applications. Dimensional analysis is useful in a wide variety of pharmaceutical calculations, as shown by the examples below. It is particularly advantageous in complex problems in which a variety of equivalents and unit-conversion factors are required. Dimensional analysis can provide, in a single equation, all of the terms required, whereas in using ratio and proportion, multiple steps and equations may be required to solve the same problem.

EXAMPLE PROBLEMS

1. How many grams of dextrose are required to prepare 4,000 mL of a 5% w/v solution? Equivalent

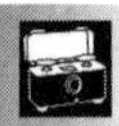

factor: a 5% w/v solution = 5 g in 100 mL of solution.

$$\frac{5\text{g}}{100\text{ mL}} \times 4{,}000\text{ mL} = 200\text{ g}$$

2. How many fluid ounces are contained in 2.5 L?

Unit-conversion factors: 1 L = 1,000 mL

1 fl oz = 29.57 mL

$$\frac{1\text{ fl oz}}{29.57\text{ mL}} \times \frac{1{,}000\text{ mL}}{1\text{ L}} \times 2.5\text{ L} = 84.5\text{ fl oz}$$

3. A medication order calls for 1,000 mL of a dextrose intravenous infusion to be administered over an 8-hour period. Using an intravenous administration set that delivers 10 drops/mL, how many drops per minute should be delivered to the patient?

$$\frac{1{,}000\text{ mL}}{8\text{ hr}} \times \frac{1\text{ hr}}{60\text{ min}} \times \frac{10\text{ drops}}{1\text{ mL}}$$

$$= 20.83\text{ drops/min} \cong 21\text{ drops/min}$$

4. The usual initial dose of chlorambucil is 150 μg/kg of body weight once per day. How many milligrams should be administered to a patient weighing 154 lb?

Unit-conversion factors: 1 mg = 1,000 μg

1 kg = 2.2 lb

$$\frac{150\ \mu\text{g}}{1\text{ kg}} \times \frac{1\text{ mg}}{1{,}000\ \mu\text{g}} \times \frac{1\text{ kg}}{2.2\text{ lb}} \times 154\text{ lb} = 10.5\text{ mg}$$

5. If an antibiotic preparation contains 5 g of penicillin V potassium in 200 mL of solution, how many milligrams of the antibiotic would be contained in each teaspoonful dose?

Unit-conversion factors: 1 gram = 1,000 mg

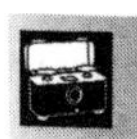

1 teaspoonful = 5 mL

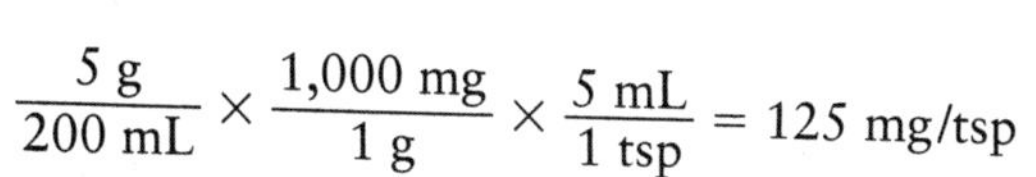

$$\frac{5\ \text{g}}{200\ \text{mL}} \times \frac{1{,}000\ \text{mg}}{1\ \text{g}} \times \frac{5\ \text{mL}}{1\ \text{tsp}} = 125\ \text{mg/tsp}$$

References

1. Ansel HC, Stoklosa MJ. Pharmaceutical Calculations. 11th Ed. Baltimore, MD: Lippincott Williams & Wilkins, 2001:13–20.
2. Craig GP. Clinical Calculations Made Easy: Solving Problems Using Dimensional Analysis. 2nd Ed. Baltimore, MD: Lippincott Williams & Wilkins, 2001.

2

SYSTEMS OF WEIGHT AND MEASUREMENT

This chapter presents the systems of weight and measurement used in pharmacy. Although the *metric system* is used almost universally nowadays, two other systems—the *apothecaries' system* and the *avoirdupois system*—have some elements of use remaining and thus are included in this chapter.

2.1 Metric System

The metric system is the internationally accepted system of weights and measures and is the official system of the *United States Pharmacopeia* (USP) and *National Formulary* (NF).[1] The metric system also is the predominant system used in writing prescriptions, medication orders, and pharmaceutical formulas.

Definition. The *metric system* is a decimal system of weights and measures.

Expressions. In the metric system, the *meter* is the primary unit of length, the *liter* of volume, and the *gram* of weight. Subdivisions and multiples of these principal units, their relative values, and their corresponding prefixes are shown in Table 2-1. The prefixes most used in

TABLE 2-1
Prefixes and Relative Values of the Metric System[a]

Prefix	Meaning
Subdivisions	
atto-	one-quintillionth (10^{-18}) of the basic unit
femto-	one-quadrillionth (10^{-15}) of the basic unit
pico-	one-trillionth (10^{-12}) of the basic unit
nano-	one-billionth (10^{-9}) of the basic unit
micro-	**one-millionth (10^{-6}) of the basic unit**
milli-	**one-thousandth (10^{-3}) of the basic unit**
centi-	**one-hundredth (10^{-2}) of the basic unit**
deci-	**one-tenth (10^{-1}) of the basic unit**
Multiples	
deka-	10 times the basic unit
hecto-	100 times (10^{2}) the basic unit
kilo-	**1000 times (10^{3}) the basic unit**
myria-	10,000 times (10^{4}) the basic unit
mega-	1 million times (10^{6}) the basic unit
giga-	1 billion times (10^{9}) the basic unit
tera-	1 trillion times (10^{12}) the basic unit
peta-	1 quadrillion times (10^{15}) the basic unit
exa-	1 quintillion times (10^{18}) the basic unit

[a] The prefixes most used in pharmacy practice are in **boldface type.**

pharmacy practice are listed in boldface type in the table.

Discussion. In this decimal-based system, the value of a number may be changed by a factor of 10 by the movement of the decimal point one position. To change a metric unit to the next smaller denomination, the decimal point is moved one place to the right. To change to the next larger denomination, the decimal point is moved one place to the left, as shown in Figure 2-1.

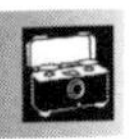

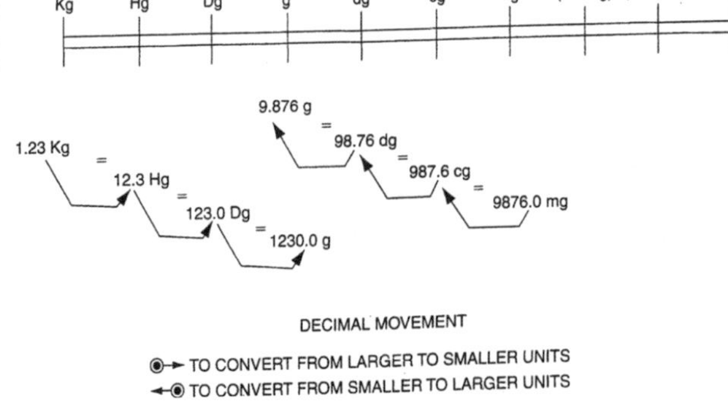

FIGURE 2-1. Metric weight scale of equivalence by decimal movement. (Reprinted with permission from Ansel HC, Stoklosa MJ. Pharmaceutical Calculations. 11th Ed. Baltimore, MD: Lippincott Williams & Wilkins, 2000:56.)

The metric units of weight and volume and their equivalents most used in pharmacy practice are:

1 milligram (mg) = 1,000 micrograms (µg or mcg)
1 gram (g) = 1,000 milligrams = 1,000,000 micrograms
1 kilogram (kg) = 1,000 grams
1 liter (L) = 1,000 milliliters (mL)
1 deciliter (dL) = 100 milliliters

In addition, the *square meter* (m^2) and the *cubic centimeter* (cm^3 or cc) often find specific application. The milliliter is so nearly the same volume as the cubic centimeter that for practical purposes they are considered equivalent units.

Although the metric system is easy to use, medication errors do occur from misplaced decimal points, incorrect unit conversions, and the unclear writing of or the misinterpretation of units. To avoid errors on prescriptions and medication orders arising from the use of an uncer-

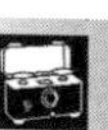

tain decimal point, a zero should be placed before the decimal point of numbers less than 1 (e.g., 0.4 mg and *NOT .4 mg*), and no zero should be placed after a whole number (e.g., 4 mg and *NOT 4.0 mg*). It should be noted, however, that in some scientific tables, compendial standards, and pharmaceutical formulas, trailing zeros *are* used to indicate the exactness of a numerical value to a certain number of decimal places. Pharmacists must be alert and check all prescriptions, medication orders, and calculations for the possibility of decimal placement errors. A misplaced decimal point leads *minimally to an error of one-tenth or 10 times the desired quantity!* In choosing among unit dimensions to express a metric quantity, the choice generally is based on the unit that results in a numeric value from 1 to 1,000. For example: 500 *g* is used rather than 0.5 *kg*; 1.96 *kg* rather than 1,960 *g*; 750 *mL* rather than 0.75 *L*; 75 *cm* rather than 0.75 *m*, and 1 *g* or 1,000 *mg* rather than 1,000,000 *μg*.

To add or subtract quantities in the metric system, all quantities must be reduced to a *common denomination* (the same unit) before engaging in the arithmetic. It is important to make certain that the decimal points are aligned to avoid errors in calculations.

EXAMPLE PROBLEMS

1. Reduce the following quantities, using Figure 2-1 as a guide.

A. 1.23 kg to grams
1.23 kg = 1,230 g

B. 9,876 mg to grams
9,876 mg = 9.876 g

C. 85 μm to centimeters
85 μm = 0.085 mm = 0.0085 cm

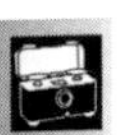

D. 2.525 L to microliters
2.525 L = 2,525 mL = 2,525,000 μL

2. If a low-strength aspirin tablet contains 81 mg of aspirin per tablet, how many tablets may be prepared from 1 kg of aspirin?

1 kg = 1,000 g = 1,000,000 mg
1,000,000 mg/81 mg = 123,456.79 ≅ 123,456 tablets

3. An inhalation aerosol contains 225 mg of metaproterenol sulfate, which is sufficient for 300 inhalations. How many micrograms of metaproterenol sulfate would be contained in each inhalation?

225 mg = 225,000 μg/300 inhalations = 750 μg

or

$$\frac{225 \text{ mg}}{300 \text{ inhalations}} \times \frac{1{,}000\ \mu\text{g}}{1 \text{ mg}} = 750\ \mu\text{g}$$

4. The following clinical laboratory data are within normal values for an adult. Convert each value to μg/mL.

A. Cholesterol (total), 150 mg/dL
150 mg = 150,000 μg
1 dL = 100 mL
150,000 μg/100 mL = 1,500 μg/mL

B. Folate, 18 pg/mL
18 pg = 0.000018 μg
0.000018 μg/mL

C. Serum creatinine, 1 mg/dL
1 mg = 1,000 μg
1 dL = 100 mL
1,000 μg/100 mL = 10 μg/mL

D. Prostate-specific antigen, 3 ng/mL
3 ng = 0.003 μg
0.003 μg/mL

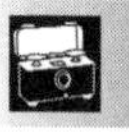

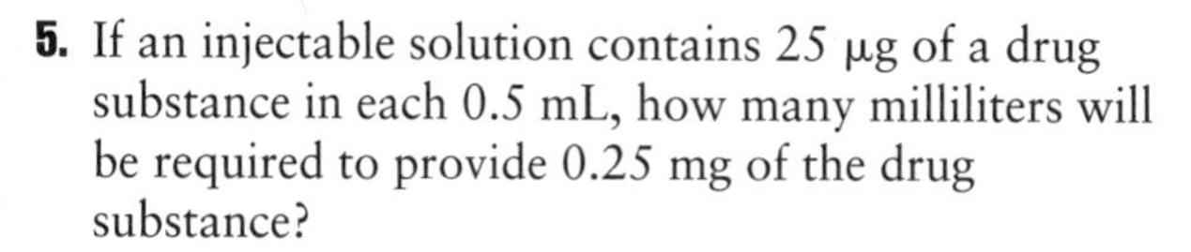

5. If an injectable solution contains 25 μg of a drug substance in each 0.5 mL, how many milliliters will be required to provide 0.25 mg of the drug substance?

$$\frac{0.5 \text{ mL}}{25 \text{ μg}} \times \frac{1{,}000 \text{ μg}}{1 \text{ mg}} \times 0.25 \text{ mg} = 5 \text{ mL}$$

6. A half-liter of D5W contains 2,000 μg of added drug. How many milliliters of the fluid would contain 0.5 mg of the drug?

$$\frac{0.5 \text{ L}}{2{,}000 \text{ μg}} \times \frac{1{,}000 \text{ mL}}{1 \text{ L}} \times \frac{1{,}000 \text{ μg}}{1 \text{ mg}} \times 0.5 \text{ mg} = 125 \text{ mL}$$

7. A solution for direct intravenous bolus injection contains 125 mg of diltiazem HCl in each 25 mL of injection. What is the concentration of diltiazem HCl in terms of μg/μL?

$$\frac{125 \text{ mg}}{25 \text{ mL}} \times \frac{1{,}000 \text{ μg}}{1 \text{ mg}} \times \frac{1 \text{ mL}}{1{,}000 \text{ μL}} = 5 \text{ μg/μL}$$

2.2 The Common Systems

The *common systems* of measurement include the apothecaries' system and the avoirdupois system. These systems have been largely replaced by the metric system; however, some components of these systems remain in use, and thus they are included in this chapter.

Definitions. The *apothecaries' system* is the traditional and historic system of weights and measures used in pharmacy. The *avoirdupois system* is the common system of commerce in which goods are purchased by weight.

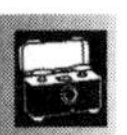

Expressions. The apothecaries' system is expressed by unique units and symbols, namely the minim (♏), grain (gr), scruple (℈), dram (ʒ), ounce (℥), and pound (℔). In contrast to the metric system, in which decimal fractions are used with the metric units, common fractions generally are used with apothecaries' units (e.g., ½ gr). When prescriptions were commonly written in the apothecaries' system, the numbers were written in Roman numerals after the denominations (e.g., ℥ iv).

The avoirdupois system uses three units of weight, the grain (gr), ounce (oz), and pound (lb). The grain has the same value of weight in both the apothecaries' and avoirdupois systems. The quantitative values of some units in the common systems are shown in Table 2-2. A complete list may be found in the referenced calculations textbook.[2]

Discussion. Among the remaining uses of the apothecaries' system are the occasional use of the dram symbol, ʒ, on prescriptions to signify a teaspoonful dose; reference to the strength of a few drugs in apothecaries' units (e.g., aspirin, 5 gr); and the common use of fluid ounce,

TABLE 2-2
Some Units in the Common Systems of Measure[a]

Measure of Weight
1 ounce (oz) = 437.5 grain (gr)
1 pound (lb) = 16 ounces

Measure of Volume
1 pint (pt) = 16 fluid ounces (fl oz or f℥)
1 quart (qt) = 2 pints
1 gallon (gal) = 4 quarts

[a] A complete list of units in the common systems may be found in *Pharmaceutical Calculations.*[2]

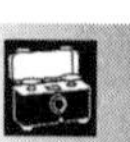

pint, quart, and gallon measures. Pharmacists must be mindful that the use of the apothecaries' system can lead to misinterpretation and error caused, for example, by the similarities between the abbreviations for grains (gr) and grams (g), and between the ʒ symbol and the Arabic numeral 3.

The pharmacist purchases bulk chemicals by the avoirdupois and/or metric systems, with some commercial packages being dual-labeled. In addition to its use in commerce, the avoirdupois system is widely used in the United States in measuring body weight. Body weight, expressed either in pounds or kilograms, is often a factor in dosage calculations, as discussed in Part C of this *Handbook*.

Key Points. If, on a metrically written prescription, the dram symbol, ʒ, is used with reference to a dose, it should be interpreted as a teaspoonful, or the equivalent of 5 mL. On the rare occasion in which a prescription is written using apothecaries' measures, those units should be converted to corresponding quantities in the metric system before further calculations. Conversion between the metric and common systems is facilitated through the use of *conversion factors*, as discussed in Section 2.3.

EXAMPLE PROBLEMS

1. How many fluid ounces are contained in 1 gallon?

$$\frac{16 \text{ fluid ounces}}{1 \text{ pint}} \times \frac{2 \text{ pints}}{1 \text{ quart}} \times \frac{4 \text{ quarts}}{1 \text{ gallon}} = 128 \text{ fluid ounces/gallon}$$

2. How many 2–fluid ounce bottles may be filled from 5 gallons of cough syrup?

$$\frac{1 \text{ bottle}}{2 \text{ fluid ounces}} \times \frac{128 \text{ fluid ounces}}{1 \text{ gallon}} \times 5 \text{ gallons} = 320 \text{ bottles}$$

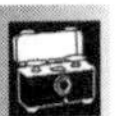

3. How many grains of a chemical remain in a 1-oz bottle after 20 gr are removed?

1 oz = 437.5 gr

437.5 gr − 20 gr = 417.5 gr

4. If a drug costs $8.75 per oz, what is the cost of 120 gr?

$$\frac{\$8.75}{1\ \text{oz}} \times \frac{1\ \text{oz}}{437.5\ \text{gr}} \times 120\ \text{gr} = \$2.40$$

5. If a chemical costs $35.00 per pound, what is the cost of 1 oz?

$$\frac{\$35.00}{1\ \text{lb}} \times \frac{1\ \text{lb}}{16\ \text{oz}} \cong \$2.19$$

2.3 Intersystem Conversion

It is sometimes necessary to convert a quantity between the metric, apothecaries', or avoirdupois systems. This is accomplished through the use of *conversion factors* or *conversion equivalents*, which provide equivalent weights and measures between the systems.

Definition. *Intersystem conversion* is the process of translating a weight or measurement from units of one system to units of another system.

Expressions. Conversion factors or conversion equivalents are expressed as shown in Table 2-3, in which a unit measure in one system has an equivalent value in another system.

Discussion. Nowadays, prescriptions and medication orders are written in the metric system, and labeling on most prefabricated pharmaceutical products has drug

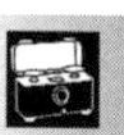

TABLE 2-3
Table of Practical Conversion Equivalents

Conversion Equivalents of Length		
1 m	=	39.37 in
1 in	=	2.54 cm
Conversion Equivalents of Volume		
1 f℥ (fluid ounce)	=	29.57 mL
1 pt	=	473 mL
1 gal (US)[a]	=	3,785 mL
1 gal (US)[a]	=	128 f℥
Conversion Equivalents of Weight		
1 g	=	15.432 gr
1 kg	=	2.20 lb
1 gr	=	0.065 g or 65 mg
1 oz (437.5 gr)	=	28.35 g
1 lb (7,000 gr)	=	454 g
Common Household Equivalents		
1 teaspoonful (tsp)	≅	5 mL
1 tablespoonful (tbsp)	≅	15 mL

[a] The US gallon is specified because the British Imperial gallon and other counterpart measures differ substantially, as follows: British Imperial gallon, 4,545 mL; pint, 568.25 mL; f℥, 28.412 mL; fʒ, 3.55 mL; and ♏, 0.059 mL. Note, however, that the metric system of weights and measures is used in both the *United States Pharmacopeia* and the *British Pharmacopoeia.*

strengths and dosages described in metric units. Manufacturing formulas and official drug standards are similarly expressed in metric units. However, on occasion it is necessary to translate quantities and units from one system of measurement to another.

The USP provides a table of *exact* equivalents of weights and measures in the metric, apothecaries', and avoirdupois systems for the conversion of specific quantities in pharmaceutical formulas.[1] The USP also pro-

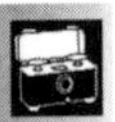

vides a table of *approximate* equivalents for the conversion of grains to milligrams.[1]

Key Points. When a high degree of precision is required in translating from one system to another, *exact conversion equivalents* rounded to three significant figures should be used. In most pharmacy practice applications, however, the approximate or practical equivalents listed in Table 2-3, with two- or three-figure accuracy, are sufficient.

A conversion factor should be selected for use that contains both the *given units* and the *units desired* (e.g., from *in* to *cm*, from *f℥* to *mL*, from *kg* to *lb*, etc.). Although any conversion factor containing both the given and the desired units is sufficient to serve as a bridge between two systems, it is sometimes prudent to select one possible conversion factor over another. For example, the factor *1 g = 15.432 gr* is useful in converting a number of *grams to grains*, but in converting *grains to grams or milligrams*, a preferred factor is *1 gr = 0.065 g or 65 mg (or more precisely, 0.0648 g or 64.8 mg)*.

For most pharmaceutical calculations, it is recommended that quantities stated in the common systems be converted to equivalent metric quantities before solving in the usual manner.

EXAMPLE PROBLEMS

1. Convert each of the following:

A. 6.35 mm to inches

$$6.35 \text{ mm} \times \frac{1 \text{ cm}}{10 \text{ mm}} \times \frac{1 \text{ in}}{2.54 \text{ cm}} = 0.25 \text{ in}$$

B. 2.5 L to fluid ounces

$$2.5 \text{ L} \times \frac{1{,}000 \text{ mL}}{1 \text{ L}} \times \frac{1 \text{ fl oz}}{29.57 \text{ mL}} = 84.545 \text{ fl oz}$$

C. 2½ pt to milliliters

$$2\tfrac{1}{2}\text{ pt} \times \frac{473\text{ mL}}{1\text{ pt}} = 1{,}182.5\text{ mL}$$

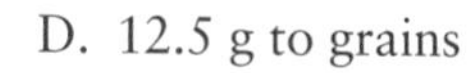

D. 12.5 g to grains

$$12.5\text{ g} \times \frac{15.432\text{ gr}}{1\text{ g}} = 192.9\text{ gr}$$

E. 15 kg to pounds

$$15\text{ kg} \times \frac{2.2\text{ lb}}{1\text{ kg}} = 33\text{ lb}$$

F. 176 lb to kilograms

$$176\text{ lb} \times \frac{1\text{ kg}}{2.2\text{ lb}} = 80\text{ kg}$$

G. 6.2 gr to milligrams

$$6.2\text{ gr} \times \frac{65\text{ mg}}{1\text{ gr}} = 403\text{ mg}$$

2. A formula for a cough syrup contains 1/8 gr of codeine phosphate per teaspoonful (5 mL). How many grams of codeine phosphate should be used in preparing 1 pint of the cough syrup?

$$\frac{1/8\text{ gr}}{5\text{ mL}} \times \frac{0.065\text{ g}}{1\text{ gr}} \times \frac{473\text{ mL}}{1\text{ pt}} = 0.769\text{ g}$$

3. A drug substance has been shown to be embryotoxic in rats at doses of 50 mg/kg/day. Express the dose on the basis of micrograms per pound per day.

$$\frac{50\text{ mg}}{1\text{ kg}} \times \frac{1{,}000\ \mu\text{g}}{1\text{ mg}} \times \frac{1\text{ kg}}{2.2\text{ lb}}$$

$$= 22{,}727.27\ \mu\text{g/lb/day}$$

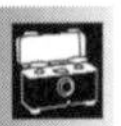

4. Tetracycline has been shown to form a calcium complex in bone-forming tissue in infants given oral tetracycline in doses of 0.011 g/lb of body weight every 6 hours. Express the dose in terms of milligrams per kilogram of body weight.

$$\frac{0.011\ \text{g}}{1\ \text{lb}} \times \frac{1{,}000\ \text{mg}}{1\ \text{g}} \times \frac{2.2\ \text{lb}}{1\ \text{kg}} = 24.2\ \text{mg/kg}$$

5. The dimensions of a nicotine transdermal patch system are 4.7 cm by 4.8 cm. Express these dimensions in corresponding inches.

$$4.7\ \text{cm} \times \frac{1\ \text{in}}{2.54\ \text{cm}} = 1.85\ \text{in, and}$$

$$4.8\ \text{cm} \times \frac{1\ \text{in}}{2.54\ \text{cm}} = 1.89\ \text{in}$$

References

1. The United States Pharmacopeia, 24th Rev., and National Formulary, 19th Ed. Rockville, MD: The United States Pharmacopeial Convention, 2000.
2. Ansel HC, Stoklosa MJ. Pharmaceutical Calculations. 11th Ed. Baltimore, MD: Lippincott Williams & Wilkins, 2001:308–309.

3

METHODS OF MEASUREMENT

Pharmacists weigh and measure pharmaceutical ingredients when called on to compound prescriptions, fill medication orders, and prepare pharmaceutical formulas, and in the manufacture and/or analysis of pharmaceuticals. This chapter describes the common methods of measurement used in pharmacy practice.

3.1 Measurement of Volume

The accurate measurement of volume is a skill acquired through a pharmacist's education and training.

Definitions. *Volume* is the space occupied as measured in cubic units. *Volumetric* relates to the measurement of volume with an appropriate instrument or device.

Discussion. Common instruments for the pharmaceutical measurement of volume range from the micropipettes and burettes used in analytic procedures to large, industrial-sized calibrated vessels. The selection of a measuring instrument should be based on the volume of material to be measured and the level of precision required. In pharmacy practice, the most common instruments for measuring volume are cylindrical and conical

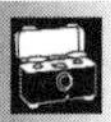

(cone-shaped) graduated vessels, and when small volumes are to be measured, calibrated syringes or pipettes.

When using a pharmaceutical graduated vessel, it is best to select one with a capacity equal to or just exceeding the volume to be measured. The measurement of small volumes in large graduated vessels increases the potential for error; the narrower the bore or chamber, the lesser the error in reading the meniscus and the more accurate the measurement (Fig. 3-1). According to the *United States Pharmacopeia*, a deviation of 1 mm in the meniscus reading causes an error of approximately 0.5 mL when a 100-mL *cylindrical* graduated vessel is used and an error of 1.8 mL at the 100-mL mark when a comparable *conical* graduated vessel is used.[1] Conical graduated vessels of less than 25-mL capacities are not recommended for use in pharmaceutical compounding.

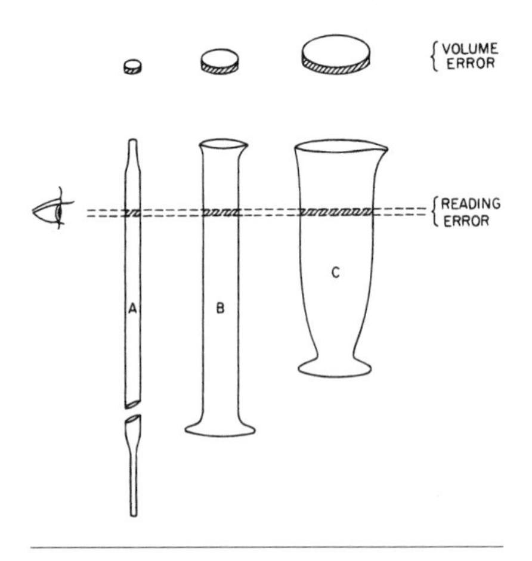

FIGURE 3-1. Volume error differentials caused by instrument diameters.

3.2 Measurement of Weight

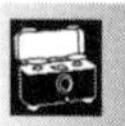

Pharmacists are uniquely qualified to accurately weigh ingredients in compounding, manufacturing, and analytic procedures.

Discussion. The selection of an instrument for the determination of weight depends on the task at hand. The choice may be made from a wide range of available instruments, including highly sensitive analytic balances, electronic or torsion prescription balances, or scales of various capacities used in the manufacture of small- and large-scale batches of pharmaceutical products. Whichever instrument is used, it must meet established standards for sensitivity, accuracy, and capacity.

Minimally, a class A prescription balance should be used in all prescription-compounding procedures. Balances of this type have a *sensitivity requirement* (SR) of 6 mg and a maximum capacity of 120 g.

If a certain percentage of error is not to be exceeded and the sensitivity of a balance is known, the smallest quantity that can be weighed within the desired accuracy may be calculated by:

$$\frac{100\% \times \text{Balance sensitivity}}{\text{Acceptable percentage of error (\%)}} = \text{Smallest quantity to be weighed}$$

Thus, for a balance with a sensitivity of 6 mg and with an acceptable error of 5%, the smallest quantity that should be weighed is 120 mg $\left(\frac{100\% \times 6\text{ mg}}{5\%} = 120\text{ mg}\right)$.

For greater precision than a class A prescription balance allows, some pharmacists use electronic balances to weigh very small quantities. Many of these balances

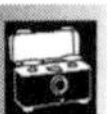

are capable of accurately weighing 0.1 mg, are self-calibrating, and are equipped with convenient digital readout features. The usual maximum capacities for balances of this precision range from about 60 g to 210 g.

EXAMPLE PROBLEM

What is the smallest quantity that can be weighed on a balance having a sensitivity requirement of 5 mg with a potential error of not more than 4%?

$$\frac{100\% \times 5 \text{ mg}}{4\%} = 125 \text{ mg}$$

3.3 Percentage of Error

An error in any measurement may occur because of the inherent sensitivity or accuracy of the instrument used and the technique applied. An error incurred may be acceptable or unacceptable depending on the degree of accuracy required. The quantification of an error is useful in assessing the procedure used.

Discussion. When a pharmacist measures a volume of liquid or weighs a material, two quantities become important in calculating the percentage of error: (1) the *apparent* weight or volume measured (*the quantity desired*), and (2) the possible excess or deficiency (*the error*) in the actual quantity obtained. In weighing, the sensitivity requirement of the balance used may constitute the error. Percentage of error may be calculated by:

$$\frac{\text{Error} \times 100\%}{\text{Quantity desired}} = \text{Percentage of error}$$

EXAMPLE PROBLEMS

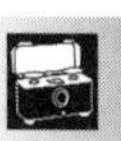

1. A pharmacist attempted to weigh 120 mg of codeine sulfate on a balance with a sensitivity requirement of 6 mg. Calculate the maximum potential error in terms of percentage.

$$\frac{6\text{ mg} \times 100\%}{120\text{ mg}} = 5\%$$

2. A pharmacist weighed 475 mg of a substance on a balance of dubious accuracy. When checked on a balance of greater accuracy, the weight was found to be 445 mg. Calculate the percentage of error in the first weighing.

$$475\text{ mg} - 445\text{ mg} = 30\text{ mg}$$

$$\frac{30\text{ mg} \times 100\%}{475\text{ mg}} = 6.3\%$$

3. Using a graduated cylinder, a pharmacist measured 30 mL of a liquid. On subsequent examination, using a narrow-gauge burette, it was determined that the pharmacist had actually measured 32 mL. What was the percentage of error in the original measurement?

$$32\text{ mL} - 30\text{ mL} = 2\text{ mL}$$

$$\frac{2\text{ mL} \times 100\%}{30\text{ mL}} = 6.7\%$$

3.4 Aliquot Method of Weighing and Measuring

When a degree of precision in measurement is required that is beyond the capacity of the instrument at hand,

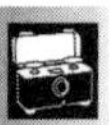

the pharmacist may achieve the desired precision by calculating and measuring in terms of aliquot parts.

Definition. An *aliquot* is a fraction, portion, or part that is contained an exact number of times in another.

Expression. An aliquot part is expressed numerically together with the same units of weight or volume as the whole (e.g., the *twentieth aliquot* of 200 g, meaning $1/20^{th}$ of 200 g).

Discussion. The aliquot method of measuring may be applied to the measurement of both weight and volume as described below. Greater detail may be found elsewhere.[2]

WEIGHING BY THE ALIQUOT METHOD

The aliquot method of weighing is a method by which small quantities of a substance may be obtained with the desired degree of accuracy by weighing a larger-than-needed portion of the substance, diluting it with an inert material, and then weighing a portion (aliquot) of the mixture calculated to contain the desired amount of the needed substance.

The aliquot method of weighing perhaps is best understood by an example, as depicted in Figure 3-2 and explained as follows.

> A prescription calls for 5 mg of a drug. A pharmacist has a prescription balance with an SR of 6 mg and accepts an error of no greater than 5% in the weighings. How would the 5 mg of drug be obtained using the aliquot method of weighing and lactose as the diluent?

The minimum weighable quantity on the balance with the accuracy desired is 120 mg $\left(\frac{100\% \times 6 \text{ mg}}{5\%} = 120 \text{ mg}\right)$.

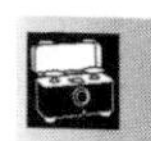

Step 1

5 mg [drug needed] × **25** [multiple factor] = 125 mg [quantity actually weighed]

Step 2

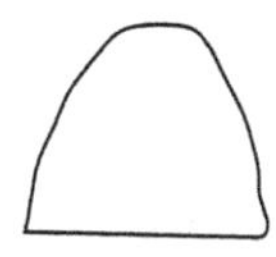

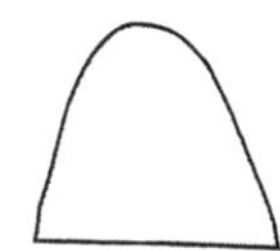

Add 2875 mg [diluent] = 3000 mg mixture [125 mg drug + 2875 mg diluent]

Step 3

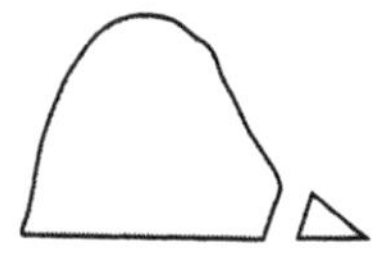

Weigh **1/25** of 3000 mg = 120 mg
[5 mg drug + 115 mg diluent]

FIGURE 3-2. Depiction of an example of the aliquot method of weighing.

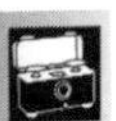

No less than this amount may be weighed throughout the procedure. The quantity of drug required, 5 mg, is obviously too little to weigh with the desired accuracy. Thus, a multiple quantity of the prescribed amount of drug must be weighed to satisfy the requirement for accuracy. A multiple factor of 25 is selected arbitrarily, and 125 mg (5 mg × 25) of drug are weighed (*step 1*). In determining the amount of lactose to add, it is important to recognize that *twenty-five times* the amount of drug that is actually needed has been weighed and thus *one-twenty-fifth* of the drug-diluent mixture must provide the 5 mg of drug required. By preparing a mixture that is 25 times the minimum weighable quantity on the balance (25 × 120 mg = 3,000 mg), the amount of lactose to add is then determined by subtraction [3,000 mg (mixture) − 125 mg (drug) = 2,875 mg (lactose)] (*step 2*). Then, after thoroughly mixing the drug and lactose, the *twenty-fifth aliquot* or $1/25^{th}$ of the mixture, equal to 120 mg, is weighed (*step 3*). It contains 5 mg of drug and 115 mg of lactose.

$$\text{Proof: } \frac{125 \text{ mg (drug)}}{3{,}000 \text{ mg (mixture)}} \times 120 \text{ mg (mixture)} = 5 \text{ mg (drug)}$$

MEASURING VOLUME BY THE ALIQUOT METHOD

The aliquot method of measuring volume may be used when relatively small volumes must be measured with increased precision when using a pharmaceutical graduated vessel. By this method, a multiple of the volume of liquid required is selected such that it achieves a *measurable amount* using the graduated vessel; that is, the volume is represented by the calibration markings or divisions on the graduated vessel. Once again, this process is best described by an example, as follows:

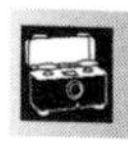

> A prescription calls for 0.5 mL of hydrochloric acid. Using a 25-mL graduated vessel calibrated in 1-mL divisions, how can the desired quantity of hydrochloric acid be obtained by the aliquot method, using water as the diluent?

If 8 is chosen as the multiple, and if 3 mL is set as the volume of the aliquot portion to contain the 0.5 mL of hydrochloric acid, then:

Measure (8 × 0.5 mL)	4 mL (acid)
Dilute with	20 mL (water)
to make (8 × 3 mL)	24 mL (dilution)

Measure 1/8 of the dilution, or 3 mL, which contains 0.5 mL of hydrochloric acid.

$$\text{Proof: } \frac{4\text{ mL (acid)}}{24\text{ mL (dilution)}} \times 3\text{ mL (dilution)} = 0.5\text{ mL (acid)}$$

Key Points. The aliquot method is a useful technique for measuring small quantities of substances in compounding procedures. It may be used when instruments with needed accuracy of measurement are unavailable. Most pharmacies that have the repeated occasion to weigh and measure small quantities should be equipped with sensitive electronic balances, pipettes, and measuring syringes.

EXAMPLE PROBLEMS

1. A torsion prescription balance has a sensitivity requirement of 6.5 mg. How would 15 mg of a drug

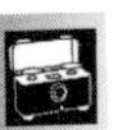

be weighed with an accuracy of 5%, using the aliquot method and lactose as the diluent?

Least weighable quantity: $\frac{100\% \times 6.5 \text{ mg}}{5\%} = 130 \text{ mg}$

Multiple factor selected: 10

Aliquot portion selected: 130 mg

Weigh (10 × 15 mg)	150 mg (drug)
Dilute with	1,150 mg (lactose)
to make (10 × 130 mg)	1,300 mg (mixture)

Weigh 1/10 of dilution, $\frac{1{,}300 \text{ mg}}{10} = 130$ mg, which contains 15 mg of drug.

2. A prescription calls for 50 mg of chlorpheniramine maleate. Using a prescription balance with a sensitivity requirement of 4 mg, explain how you would obtain the required amount of chlorpheniramine maleate with an error not greater than 4%.

Least weighable quantity: $\frac{100\% \times 4 \text{ mg}}{4\%} = 100 \text{ mg}$

Multiple factor selected: 2

Aliquot portion selected: 100 mg

Weigh (2 × 50 mg)	100 mg (drug)
Dilute with	100 mg (lactose)
to make (2 × 100 mg)	200 mg (mixture)

Weigh 1/2 of dilution, or 100 mg, which contains 50 mg of chlorpheniramine maleate.

3. A prescription calls for 0.2 mL of clove oil. Using a 25-mL graduated vessel calibrated in units of 0.5 mL, how would you obtain the required amount of

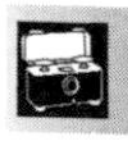

clove oil using the aliquot method and alcohol as the diluent?

Aliquot chosen: 2 mL

Multiple chosen: 10

Measure (10 × 0.2 mL)	2 mL (clove oil)
Dilute with	18 mL (alcohol)
to make (10 × 2 mL)	20 mL (dilution)

Measure 1/10 of the dilution, or 2 mL, which contains 0.2 mL of clove oil.

4. A pharmaceutical formula calls for 0.4 mL of the surfactant polysorbate 80. Using water as the diluent and a 25-mL graduated vessel calibrated in 1-mL units, how could you obtain the desired quantity of polysorbate 80 by the aliquot method using water as the diluent?

Aliquot chosen: 4 mL

Multiple chosen: 10

Measure (10 × 0.4 mL)	4 mL (polysorbate 80)
Dilute with	16 mL (water)
to make	20 mL (dilution)

Measure 1/10 of the dilution, or 2 mL, which contains 0.4 mL of polysorbate 80.

References

1. The United States Pharmacopeia. 24th Rev. and National Formulary, 19th Ed. Rockville, MD: United States Pharmacopeial Convention, 2000.
2. Ansel HC, Stoklosa MJ. Pharmaceutical Calculations. 11th Ed. Baltimore, MD: Lippincott Williams & Wilkins, 2001.

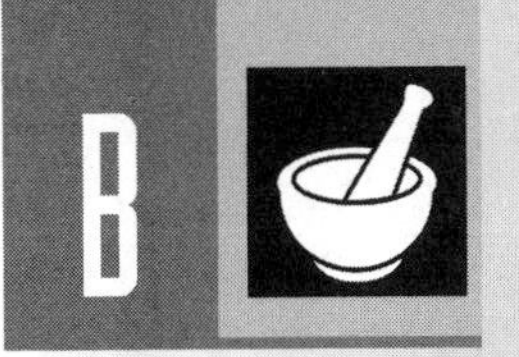

Prescription Compounding and Formulation Calculations

CHAPTER 9 Isotonic Solutions

9.1 The Dissociation Factor of an Electrolyte
9.2 Sodium Chloride Equivalents
9.3 Preparation of Isotonic Solutions

CHAPTER 10 Electrolyte Solutions

10.1 Milliequivalents
10.2 Millimoles
10.3 Milliosmoles and Osmolarity

4

EXPRESSIONS OF CONCENTRATION

This chapter presents expressions of concentration most commonly encountered in the practice of pharmacy.

4.1 Percentage Strength

Percentage strength is used in pharmacy practice as a convenient means of expressing the concentration of an active or inactive material in a pharmaceutical preparation.

Definitions. The term *percent* and its corresponding sign, %, mean "by the hundred" or "in a hundred," and *percentage* means "*rate* per hundred." Qualifying definitions of the percentage strength of pharmaceutical preparations, based on their composition, are contained in the *United States Pharmacopeia*[1] (USP) as indicated by the following expressions.

Expressions. The percentage strengths of pharmaceutical preparations are expressed as follows, with the first term (or numerator) of each expression indicating the component on which the strength of the preparation is based and the second term (or denominator) indicating the preparation as a whole.

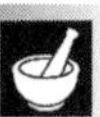

- *Percent weight-in-volume* (w/v) expresses the number of *grams* of a constituent in *100 mL* of solution or liquid preparation, and is used regardless of whether water or another liquid is the solvent or vehicle. Expressed as: ___ % *w/v.*
- *Percent volume-in-volume* (v/v) expresses the number of *milliliters* of a constituent in *100 mL* of solution or liquid preparation. Expressed as: ___ % *v/v.*
- *Percent weight-in-weight* (w/w) expresses the number of *grams* of a constituent in *100 g* of solution or preparation. Expressed as: ___ % *w/w.*

Discussion. Often on prescriptions and in formulas, the designations w/v, v/v, and w/w are not indicated when percentage strengths are given. In these instances, the following is assumed:

- For solutions or dispersions of solids in liquids, *percent weight-in-volume*;
- For solutions or dispersions of liquids in liquids, *percent volume-in-volume*;
- For mixtures of solids or semisolids, *percent weight-in-weight*; and
- For solutions of gases in liquids, *percent weight-in-volume.*

In multiple-ingredient prescriptions or formulas, it is not unusual for one ingredient to be calculated on a w/v basis and another on a v/v basis. For example, in compounding a liquid preparation, one ingredient may be a powder and calculated on a w/v basis and another ingredient may be a liquid and calculated on a v/v basis.

In calculations, percents may be expressed as ratios, indicating parts per hundred, for example, 5% may be restated as $\frac{5}{100}$, or they may be changed to equivalent

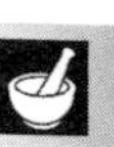

decimal fractions by dropping the percent sign and dividing the number by *100*. Thus, *5%* = 5 ÷ 100 = 0.05, *12.5%* = 12.5 ÷ 100 = 0.125, and *0.05%* = 0.05 ÷ 100 = 0.0005. In the reverse process, to change a decimal fraction to a percent, the decimal fraction is multiplied by *100* and the percent sign added. For example, 0.125 × 100 = 12.5%.

Key Points. It is important to define the basis on which a pharmaceutical calculation is to be performed (i.e., w/v, v/v, or w/w) to have the units of the calculation correct. Pharmaceutical calculations involving percentage strength are generally of two types: (1) the percentage strength of an active or inactive component in a prescription or formula is stated, and the *quantity of the needed ingredient is to be determined*, and (2) the quantity of an active or inactive ingredient in a prescription or formula is stated, and its *percent concentration in the preparation is to be determined.*

Pharmacy Applications. Percentage strength is a standard measure of the concentration of a component in a pharmaceutical preparation. In fact, the concentration of most pharmaceutical products may be described in terms of percentage strength. In the example problems that follow, problems 1 through 8 demonstrate weight-in-volume calculations; 9 and 10 demonstrate volume-in-volume calculations; and 11 through 13 demonstrate weight-in-weight calculations.

EXAMPLE PROBLEMS

Weight-in-Volume

1. What is the percentage strength of an injection that contains 50 mg of pentobarbital sodium in each milliliter of solution?

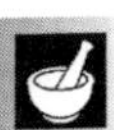

$$\frac{50 \text{ mg}}{1 \text{ mL}} \times \frac{1 \text{ g}}{1{,}000 \text{ mg}} \times 100 = 5\% \text{ w/v}$$

2. The biotechnology-derived product Neupogen contains 300 μg of filgrastim in each milliliter of injection. Calculate the percent concentration of filgrastim in the product.

$$\frac{300 \text{ μg}}{1 \text{ mL}} \times \frac{1 \text{ g}}{1{,}000{,}000 \text{ μg}} \times 100 = 0.03\% \text{ w/v}$$

3. If an injection contains 0.5% w/v of diltiazem hydrochloride, calculate the number of milligrams of the drug in 25 mL of injection.

$$\frac{0.5 \text{ g}}{100 \text{ mL}} \times \frac{1{,}000 \text{ mg}}{1 \text{ g}} \times 25 \text{ mL} = 125 \text{ mg}$$

4. How many grams of potassium permanganate should be used in compounding the following prescription?

℞	Potassium permanganate	0.02% w/v
	Purified water ad	250 mL

$$\frac{0.02 \text{ g}}{100 \text{ mL}} \times 250 \text{ mL} = 0.05 \text{ g}$$

5. A pharmacist adds 10 mL of a 20% w/v solution of potassium iodide to 500 mL of D5W for parenteral infusion. What is the percentage strength of potassium iodide in the infusion solution?

Total volume of solution

$$= 500 \text{ mL} + 10 \text{ mL} = 510 \text{ mL}$$

$$10 \text{ mL} \times \frac{20 \text{ g}}{100 \text{ mL}} = 2 \text{ g (potassium iodide)}$$

$$\frac{2 \text{ g}}{510 \text{ mL}} \times 100 = 0.39\% \text{ w/v}$$

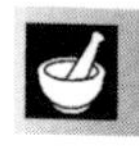

6. ℞ Misoprostol 200-μg tablets 12 tablets
Lidocaine hydrochloride 1 g
Glycerin qs ad 100 mL

Calculate the percent strength of misoprostol in the prescription.

$200\ \mu g \times 12\ (\text{tablets}) = 2{,}400\ \mu g$

$$\frac{2{,}400\ \mu g}{100\ mL} \times \frac{1 g}{1{,}000{,}000\ \mu g} \times 100 = 0.0024\%\ w/v$$

7. How many liters of a 2% w/v iodine tincture can be made from 123 g of iodine?

$$\frac{100\ mL}{2\ g} \times \frac{1\ L}{1{,}000\ mL} \times 123\ g = 6.15\ L$$

8. ℞[2] Gentamicin (40 mg/mL) injection 2 mL
Gentamicin (0.3%) ophthalmic solution 5 mL

Calculate the percent concentration of gentamicin in this fortified ophthalmic solution.

Total volume of solution = 7 mL

$$\frac{40\ mg}{1\ mL} \times \frac{1\ g}{1{,}000\ mg} \times 2\ mL = 0.08\ g, \text{ and}$$

$$\frac{0.3\ g}{100\ mL} \times 5\ mL = 0.015\ g, \text{ then}$$

$$0.08\ g + 0.015\ g = 0.095\ g, \text{ and}$$

$$\frac{0.095\ g}{7\ mL} \times 100\ mL = 1.36\%\ w/v$$

Volume-in-Volume

9. One gallon of a certain lotion contains 946 mL of benzyl benzoate. Calculate the percentage strength (v/v) of benzyl benzoate in the lotion.

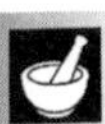

$$\frac{946 \text{ mL}}{1 \text{ gallon}} \times \frac{1 \text{ gallon}}{3{,}785 \text{ mL}} \times 100 = 24.99\% \text{ v/v}$$

10. How many milliliters of liquefied phenol should be used in compounding the following prescription?

℞		
	Liquefied phenol	2.5%
	Calamine lotion ad	240 mL

$2.5\% = 0.025$

$240 \text{ mL} \times 0.025 = 6 \text{ mL}$

or

$$\frac{2.5 \text{ mL}}{100 \text{ mL}} \times 240 \text{ mL} = 6 \text{ mL}$$

Weight-in-Weight

11. ℞

Iodochlorhydroxyquin	0.9 g
Hydrocortisone	0.15 g
Cream base ad	30 g

What is the percentage strength (w/w) each of iodochlorhydroxyquin and hydrocortisone in the prescription?

$$\frac{0.9 \text{ g}}{30 \text{ g}} \times 100 = 3\% \text{ w/w, iodochlorhydroxyquin}$$

$$\frac{0.15 \text{ g}}{30 \text{ g}} \times 100 = 0.5\% \text{ w/w, hydrocortisone}$$

12. How many milligrams of procaine hydrochloride should be used in preparing 120 suppositories each weighing 2 g and containing 1/4% of procaine hydrochloride?

$2 \text{ g} \times 120 \text{ (suppositories)} = 240 \text{ g}$

$1/4\% = 0.25\%$

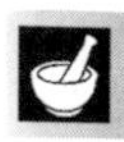

$$\frac{0.25\ g}{100\ g} \times \frac{1{,}000\ mg}{1\ g} \times 240\ g = 600\ mg$$

13. How many grams of a drug substance should be *added to* 240 mL of water to make a 4% (w/w) solution?

100% − 4% = 96% (the water component in the final preparation)

240 mL of water weighs 240 g

$$\frac{4\ g}{96\ g} \times 240\ g = 10\ g$$

Proof: 10 g + 240 g = 250 g

$$\frac{10\ g}{250\ g} \times 100 = 4\%\ w/w$$

Weight-in-Volume/Volume-in-Volume

14. ℞

Resin of podophyllum	25%
Tolu balsam tincture	5%
Compound benzoin tincture ad 30 mL	

How many grams of resin of podophyllum and milliliters of tolu balsam tincture should be used in preparing the prescription?

$$\frac{25\ g}{100\ mL} \times 30\ mL = 7.5\ g\text{, resin of podophyllum}$$

$$\frac{5\ mL}{100\ mL} \times 30\ mL = 1.5\ mL\text{, tolu balsam tincture}$$

4.2 Ratio Strength

The concentrations of pharmaceutical preparations may be expressed in terms of ratio strength.

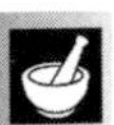

Definition. *Ratio strength* expresses, in the form of a ratio, the concentration of an agent relative to the total preparation.

Expression. Ratio strengths are expressed as a ratio of two numbers, separated by a colon as shown by the examples below. The number to the left of the colon represents the relative quantity of the substance whose strength is being defined, and the number to the right of the colon represents the quantity of the total preparation. A qualifying designation of the type of pharmaceutical preparation (i.e., v/v, w/v, or w/w) may or may not be included with the ratio strength. If it is not, the type of preparation is assumed, based on its physical composition.

Examples: 1:1,000 or 1:1,000 v/v
1:15,000 or 1:15,000 w/v
3:200 or 3:200 w/w

Ratio strengths are read, as in the examples:

"1 part in 1,000 parts," "1 in 1,000," or "1 mL in 1,000 mL"
"1 part in 15,000 parts," "1 in 15,000," or "1 g in 15,000 mL"
"3 parts in 200 parts," "3 in 200," or "3 g in 200 g"

Discussion. Ratio strength and percentage strength both involve the concept of ratios. Percentage strength, by definition, relates parts per hundred. For example, *5%* means *5 parts per 100* or the ratio *5:100*. Unlike percentage strength, which is based on parts per 100, ratio strength is not used on any set numerical base. Ratio strengths usually are used to express the concentration of very dilute preparations and most often are stated in terms of the whole number 1 preceding the colon (e.g., 1:10,000; 1:15,000, 1:40,000).

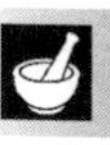

When a ratio strength, for example *1:1,000*, is used to designate a concentration without an accompanying designation of the type of preparation (i.e., v/v, w/v, or w/w), it is interpreted as follows, based on its components:

- *For solids in liquids* = *1 g* of solute or constituent in *1,000 mL* of solution or liquid preparation
- *For liquids in liquids* = *1 mL* of constituent in *1,000 mL* of solution or liquid preparation
- *For solids in solids* = *1 g* of constituent in *1,000 g* of mixture

A calculations problem may be solved directly using a given ratio strength, or the ratio strength may be converted to the corresponding percentage strength and the problem may be solved on that basis. The ratio and proportion method of calculations (see Chapter 1) often is preferred for solving problems of ratio strength. When seeking a ratio strength, a proportion may be set up with the number 1 in the numerator and x in the denominator, so that in solving for x the answer yields a ratio strength of 1:x (the numerical answer). For example:

If there are 50 mg of drug in 1 liter of solution, calculate the solution's ratio strength, w/v.

Because ratio strength w/v is defined in terms of g/mL, we must change:

50 mg = 0.05 g

1 L = 1,000 mL

then, by proportion:

$$\frac{0.05\text{ g}}{1{,}000\text{ mL}} = \frac{1}{x}; \; 0.05x = 1{,}000; \; x = 20{,}000$$

Thus, there is the equivalent of 1 g in 20,000 mL, or a ratio strength of 1:20,000 w/v.

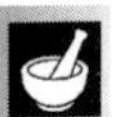

Ratio strengths can be converted to percentage strengths and vice versa as shown by the following examples:

Express 0.02% as a ratio strength.

0.02% = 0.02 parts per 100 parts

Then, solving by proportion to yield a ratio strength of 1:_____

$$\frac{0.02}{100} = \frac{1}{x}; \; 0.02x = 100; \; x = \frac{100}{0.02}; \; x = 5{,}000$$

Ratio strength = 1:5,000
Alternatively, 100 ÷ 0.02 = 5,000; and thus the ratio strength of 1:5,000

Express 1:4,000 as a percentage strength.

By setting up and solving the following proportion, the answer to "x" will result in parts per 100 and thus, by definition, the percentage strength.

$$\frac{1}{4{,}000} = \frac{x}{100}; \; 4{,}000x = 100; \; x = \frac{100}{4{,}000};$$

$$x = 0.025\%$$

Alternatively, 1 ÷ 4,000 = 0.00025; or the percentage strength of 0.025%

To change ratio strength to percent strength, it is sometimes convenient to "convert" the last two zeros in a ratio strength to a percent sign (%), and change the remaining ratio to a common fraction, and then to a decimal fraction in expressing percent. For example, 1:4,000 can be interpreted as 1/40% or 0.025%.

Key Point. Whenever arithmetically possible, it is best to reduce a ratio strength such that the ingredient whose

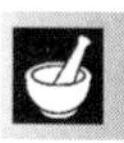

strength is being expressed is stated as 1, such as 1:250 rather than 4:1,000. When this is not feasible, a ratio strength such as 3:200 would be preferred over one with a decimal fraction, such as 1:66.67.

Pharmacy Applications. In pharmacy practice, ratio strengths are used for convenience to express the strength of very dilute preparations (e.g., 1:20,000), rather than using equivalent decimal fractions (e.g., 0.005%).

EXAMPLE PROBLEMS

1. A certain injectable contains 2 mg of a drug per milliliter of solution. What is the ratio strength and the corresponding percentage strength of the solution?

2 mg = 0.002 g

$$\frac{0.002\ (\text{g})}{1\ (\text{mL})} = \frac{1\ (\text{g})}{\text{x}\ (\text{mL})};\ 0.002\text{x} = 1;\ \text{x} = 500$$

Ratio strength = 1:500 w/v

$$\frac{0.002\ \text{g}}{1\ \text{mL}} \times 100 = 0.2\%\ \text{w/v, percentage strength}$$

2. A sample of white petrolatum contains 10 mg of tocopherol per kilogram as a preservative. Express the amount of tocopherol as a ratio strength.

10 mg = 0.01 g

1 kg = 1,000 g

$$\frac{0.01\ (\text{g})}{1{,}000\ (\text{g})} = \frac{1}{\text{x}};\ 0.01\ \text{x} = 1{,}000;\ \text{x} = 100{,}000$$

Ratio strength = 1:100,000 w/w

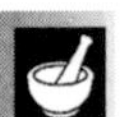

3. An ophthalmic solution of sulfacetamide sodium is preserved with 0.0008% w/v of phenylmercuric acetate. Express this concentration as a ratio strength.

$$\frac{0.0008\ (g)}{100\ (mL)} = \frac{1\ (g)}{x\ (mL)};\ 0.0008\ x = 100;\ x = 125{,}000$$

Ratio strength = 1:125,000 w/v

4. ℞ Potassium permanganate tablets 0.2 g/tab

Disp. #100 tablets

Sig. Dissolve 2 tablets in sufficient water to prepare 4 pints of solution. Use as a soak externally as directed.

Calculate the ratio strength of the solution prepared according to the directions.

$$2\ (tablets) \times 0.2\ g = 0.4\ g$$

$$4\ pt \times \frac{473\ mL}{1\ pt} = 1{,}892\ mL$$

$$\frac{0.4\ (g)}{1{,}892\ (mL)} = \frac{1}{x};\ 0.4x = 1{,}892;\ x = 4{,}730$$

Ratio strength = 1:4,730 w/v

5. For bladder and urethral irrigation, it is recommended to dilute each 3 mL of a 1:750 w/v solution of benzalkonium chloride with 77 mL of sterile water. What is the ratio strength of benzalkonium chloride in the resultant solution?

Total volume of solution = 80 mL

$$\frac{1\ g}{750\ mL} \times 3\ mL = 0.004\ g\ \text{benzalkonium chloride}$$

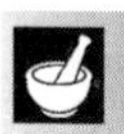

$$\frac{0.004 \text{ (g)}}{80 \text{ (mL)}} = \frac{1}{x}; 0.004\ x = 80; x = 20{,}000$$

Ratio strength = 1:20,000 w/v

6. How many grams of potassium permanganate should be used in preparing 500 mL of a 1:2,500 solution?

$$\frac{1 \text{ g}}{2{,}500 \text{ mL}} \times 500 \text{ mL} = 0.2 \text{ g}$$

7. How many milligrams of gentian violet should be used in preparing the following prescription?

℞ Gentian violet solution (1:10,000) 500 mL
Sig. Use externally as directed.

$$\frac{1 \text{ g}}{10{,}000 \text{ mL}} \times 500 \text{ mL} = 0.05 \text{ g} = 50 \text{ mg}$$

4.3 Milligrams Percent

Milligrams percent is a way of expressing the concentration of small quantities of a substance, usually in a biologic fluid.

Definition. *Milligrams percent* expresses the number of milligrams of substance in 100 mL of liquid.

Expression. *Milligrams percent* is expressed as *mg%*.

Discussion. *Milligrams percent* is used frequently to denote the concentration of a drug or natural substance in a biologic fluid such as blood. For example, the statement that the concentration of nonprotein nitrogen in the blood is 30 mg% means that each 100 mL of blood

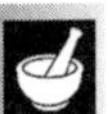

contains 30 mg of nonprotein nitrogen. The quantities of substances present in biologic fluids also commonly are stated in terms of milligrams per deciliter (mg/dL) of fluid. Because 1 dL equals 100 mL, the value of a specific quantity expressed in mg% would be the same when expressed in mg/dL.

EXAMPLE PROBLEMS

1. If a patient is determined to have a serum cholesterol level of 200 mg/dL, (A) what is the equivalent value expressed in terms of milligrams percent, and (B) how many milligrams of cholesterol would be present in a 10-mL sample of the patient's serum?

A. 200 mg/dL = 200 mg/100 mL = 200 mg%

B. $$\frac{200\ \text{mg}}{1\ \text{dL}} \times \frac{1\ \text{dL}}{100\ \text{mL}} = 200\ \text{mg}/100\ \text{mL}$$

$$= 20\ \text{mg}/10\ \text{mL}$$

2. A glucose meter shows that a patient's blood contains 125 mg% of glucose. Express this value as mg/mL.

125 mg% = 125 mg/100 mL = 1.25 mg/mL

3. Federal rules prohibit transportation workers from performing safety-sensitive functions when breath alcohol level is 0.04% w/v or greater. Express this value as mg/dL.

0.04% w/v = 0.04 g/100 mL

= 40 mg/100 mL = 40 mg/dL

or

$$\frac{0.04\ \text{g}}{100\ \text{mL}} \times \frac{1{,}000\ \text{mg}}{1\ \text{g}} \times \frac{100\ \text{mL}}{1\ \text{dL}} = 40\ \text{mg/dL}$$

4.4 Parts per Million and Parts per Billion

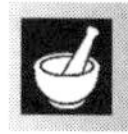

The strengths of extremely dilute solutions may be expressed in *parts per million (ppm)* or *parts per billion (ppb)*.

Definition. The terms *parts per million (ppm)* and *parts per billion (ppb)* quantify the number of parts of the agent per 1 million or 1 billion parts of the whole.

Expressions. *Parts per million* and *parts per billion* are expressed most commonly as whole numbers or decimal fractions followed by the abbreviations *ppm* or *ppb* (e.g., 10 ppm, 0.5 ppb). The usual interpretations would apply for w/v, v/v, and w/w situations; for example, *ppm w/v* indicates grams of substance in 1 million mL of solution.

Discussion. Measuring or expressing the concentration of a substance in parts per million or parts per billion occurs in a limited number of instances. One well-known example is fluoridated drinking water, in which the fluoride content is expressed in terms of parts of fluoride per million parts of drinking water (usually 1 ppm). Another example is the measurement and expression in parts per million or billion of trace quantities of substances in chemical or environmental samples.

EXAMPLE PROBLEMS

1. Express 5 ppm of iron in water as a ratio strength and in percentage strength.

5 ppm = 5 parts in 1,000,000 parts

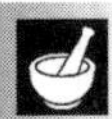

Ratio strength: 5:1,000,000 = 1:200,000

Percent strength: $\frac{5}{1,000,000} \times 100 = 0.0005\%$

2. The concentration of a drug additive in an animal feed is 12.5 ppm. How many milligrams of the drug should be used in preparing 5.2 kg of feed?

12.5 ppm = 12.5 g (drug) in 1,000,000 g (feed)

$$\frac{12.5 \text{ g}}{1,000,000 \text{ g}} \times \frac{1,000 \text{ g}}{1 \text{ kg}} \times \frac{1,000 \text{ mg}}{1 \text{ g}} \times 5.2 \text{ kg} = 65 \text{ mg}$$

3. Purified water contains not more than 10 ppm of total solids. Express this concentration as a percent.

$$\frac{10}{1,000,000} \times 100 = 0.001\%$$

4. How many grams of sodium fluoride should be added to 100,000 L of drinking water containing 0.6 ppm of sodium fluoride to provide a recommended concentration of 1.75 ppm?

$$\frac{0.6 \text{ g}}{1,000,000 \text{ mL}} \times \frac{1,000 \text{ mL}}{1 \text{ L}} \times 100,000 \text{ L} = 60 \text{ g}$$

$$\frac{1.75 \text{ g}}{1,000,000 \text{ mL}} \times \frac{1,000 \text{ mL}}{1 \text{ L}} \times 100,000 \text{ L} = 175 \text{ g}$$

175 g − 60 g = 115 g

5. If a commercially available insulin preparation contains 1 ppm of proinsulin, how many micrograms of proinsulin would be contained in a 10-mL vial of insulin?

$$\frac{1 \text{ g}}{1,000,000 \text{ mL}} \times \frac{1,000,000 \ \mu\text{g}}{1 \text{ g}} \times 10 \text{ mL} = 10 \ \mu\text{g}$$

4.5 Units, μg/mg, and Other Measures of Potency

The potency of some antibiotics, endocrine products, vitamins, and biologics (e.g., vaccines) is based on their demonstrated biologic *activity* and is expressed by various terms of measurement as described below. These measures of potency meet standards approved by the U.S. Food and Drug Administration and are set forth in the USP.[1]

Definition. The designation *USP unit(s)*, when used in conjunction with a specific agent, is a measure of that agent's potency based on standardized tests of its biologic activity. When agents conform to established international standards of potency, they are defined by the term *international unit(s) (IU)*. In some instances, biologic activity is defined in terms of weight, as *micrograms* (of active agent) *per milligram*, or by other terms and standards of measure.

Expressions. Expressions of biologic potency vary depending on the specific agent or type of agent. *Units* of biologic activity generally are expressed for certain antibiotics and hormones. The strengths of bacterial vaccines commonly are stated in *micrograms* or *units of antigen per milliliter (μg/mL* or *units/mL.)* Viral vaccines often are expressed in terms of the *tissue culture infectious dose* ($TCID_{50}$), which is the quantity of virus estimated to infect 50% of inoculated cultures. The strengths of viral vaccines may also be described in terms of *units*, *micrograms of antigen*, or the *number of organisms per milliliter*. Toxoids generally are expressed in terms of *flocculating units (Lf)*, with 1 Lf having the capacity to flocculate or precipitate 1 unit of standard antitoxin.

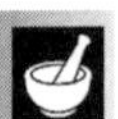

Discussion. Measure of activity is determined by comparison with a suitable working standard, generally a USP reference standard. Reference standards are authentic specimens used as comparison standards in compendial tests and assays. The number of *USP units* of an antibiotic, for example, is based on a comparison of activity of a sample of that antibiotic to the corresponding USP reference standard. Most biologic products are allowed specific variances in potency; for example, the USP monograph for sterile penicillin G sodium specifies a potency of not less than 1,500 penicillin G units and not more than 1,750 penicillin G units per milligram.[1] The activity or potency of antibiotics is determined by their inhibitory effect on microorganisms. The potency of some antibiotics may be designated in terms of micrograms of activity. For example, ampicillin sodium has a potency equivalent from 845 to 988 μg/mg of its parent compound ampicillin.[1] No relationship exists between the specific units of potency of one drug and the units of potency of another drug. Table 4-1 presents some examples of official drug potencies expressed either in units or on a weight basis.

Of the drugs for which potency is expressed in units, insulin, heparin, and the penicillin antibiotics are perhaps the most common. In the case of insulin, although the commercially available types vary according to time of onset of action, time of peak action, and duration of action, all products are standardized to contain either 100 or 500 insulin units per milliliter of solution or suspension. These package strengths are designated as U-100 and U-500. Special syringes are available for measuring units of insulin, and the required dosage is then measured in milliliters, or directly in units, depending on the calibration of the syringe. Figure 4-1 shows an example of a dual-scale insulin syringe.

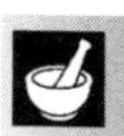

TABLE 4-1
Examples of Terms of Drug Potency

Drug	Units or μg of Potency by Weight[a]
Ampicillin sodium	NLT 845 μg and NMT 988 μg of ampicillin per mg
Antihemophilic factor	NLT 100 antihemophilic factor units per g of protein
Bacitracin	NLT 40 bacitracin units per mg
Clindamycin hydrochloride	NLT 800 μg of clindamycin per mg
Cod liver oil	NLT 255 μg (850 USP units) of vitamin A and NLT 2.125 μg (85 USP units) of vitamin D per g
Erythromycin estolate	NLT 600 μg of erythromycin per mg
Gentamicin sulfate	NLT 590 μg of gentamicin per mg
Heparin sodium	NLT 140 USP heparin units per mg
Insulin	NLT 26.5 USP insulin units per mg
Insulin human	NLT 27.5 USP insulin human units per mg
Penicillin G potassium	NLT 1,440 and NMT 1,680 penicillin G units per mg
Polymyxin B sulfate	NLT 6,000 polymyxin B units per mg
Tobramycin	NLT 900 μg of tobramycin per mg
Vitamin A	1 USP vitamin A unit equals the biologic activity of 0.3 μg of the all-trans isomer of retinol

[a] Examples taken from the United States Pharmacopeia.[1]

NLT, not less than; NMT, not more than.

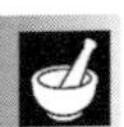

FIGURE 4-1. Example of a dual-scale insulin syringe. (Courtesy of Becton-Dickinson and Company.)

In some instances, the blood or blood serum levels of certain drugs may be expressed in the literature as mU/mL, meaning *milliunits* of the agent per milliliter of blood or blood serum.

Key Points. The terms used to describe the potency of biologic products vary depending on the specific product. Thus, pharmacists must know the specific standard of potency and dosage applicable to each product and must understand that with the term *units*, no cross-relationship exists between the units of potency of one drug and the units of potency of another drug.

To avoid possible dispensing errors, it is good practice not to abbreviate the term *units* when writing or transcribing a prescription. A poorly written U can be mistaken for a trailing zero (e.g., "insulin 100 U" may be mistakenly read as "insulin 1,000").

EXAMPLE PROBLEMS

1. How many milliliters of a package labeled "U-100 insulin" should be used to obtain 40 units of insulin?

U-100 insulin contains 100 units/mL

$$\frac{1 \text{ mL}}{100 \text{ units}} \times 40 \text{ units} = 0.4 \text{ mL}$$

2. How many milliliters of a heparin sodium injection containing 200,000 heparin units in 10 mL should be used to obtain 5,000 heparin units?

$$\frac{10\text{ mL}}{200{,}000\text{ units}} \times 5{,}000\text{ units} = 0.25\text{ mL}$$

3. A biologic contains 50 Lf units of diphtheria toxoid in each 2.5 mL of product. If a pediatric patient is to receive 10 Lf units, how many milliliters of product should be administered?

$$\frac{2.5\text{ mL}}{50\text{ Lf units}} \times 10\text{ Lf units} = 0.5\text{ mL}$$

4. Measles virus vaccine live is prepared to contain 1,000 $TCID_{50}$ per 0.5-mL dose. What is the $TCID_{50}$ content of a 50-mL multiple-dose vial of the vaccine?

$$\frac{1{,}000\text{ TCID}_{50}}{0.5\text{ mL}} \times 50\text{ mL} = 100{,}000\text{ TCID}_{50}$$

5. The biotechnology-derived product interferon beta-1b contains 32 million IU per milligram. Calculate the number of international units present in a vial containing 0.3 mg of interferon beta-1b.

$$\frac{32{,}000{,}000\text{ IU}}{1\text{ mg}} \times 0.3\text{ mg} = 9{,}600{,}000\text{ IU}$$

6. A physician prescribes 60 mL of phenoxymethyl penicillin for oral suspension containing 4,800,000 units. How many penicillin units will be represented in each teaspoonful dose of the prepared suspension?

$$\frac{4{,}800{,}000\text{ units}}{60\text{ mL}} \times 5\text{ mL} = 400{,}000\text{ units}$$

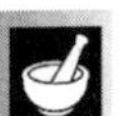

7. If 10 μg of ergocalciferol represent 400 units of vitamin D, how many 1.25-mg ergocalciferol capsules will provide a dose of 200,000 units of vitamin D?

$$\frac{10\ \mu g}{400\ units} \times \frac{1\ mg}{1{,}000\ \mu g} \times \frac{1\ capsule}{1.25\ mg} \times 200{,}000\ units = 4\ capsules$$

8. Corticotropin injection is available in a concentration of 40 units/mL. How many milliliters of the injection should be administered to provide 0.4 unit/kg for a child weighing 66 lb?

$$\frac{1\ mL}{40\ units} \times \frac{0.4\ unit}{1\ kg} \times \frac{1\ kg}{2.2\ lb} \times 66\ lb = 0.3\ mL$$

9. A physician's hospital medication order calls for 0.5 mL of U-500 insulin injection to be placed in a 500-mL bottle of 5% dextrose injection for infusion into a patient. If the infusion was set to run for 8 hours, how many units of insulin did the patient receive in the first 90 minutes of infusion?

$$0.5\ mL \times 500\ units/mL = 250\ units$$

$$\frac{250\ units}{500\ mL} \times \frac{500\ mL}{8\ hr} \times \frac{1\ hr}{60\ min} \times 90\ min = 46.88\ units$$

10. Using Table 4.1, calculate the clindamycin potency equivalence, in milligrams per milliliter, of a solution containing 1 g of clindamycin hydrochloride in 10 mL of solution.

$$\frac{1\ g}{10\ mL} \times \frac{1{,}000\ mg}{1\ g} \times \frac{800\ \mu g}{1\ mg} \times \frac{1\ mg}{1{,}000\ \mu g} = 80\ mg/mL$$

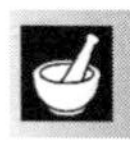

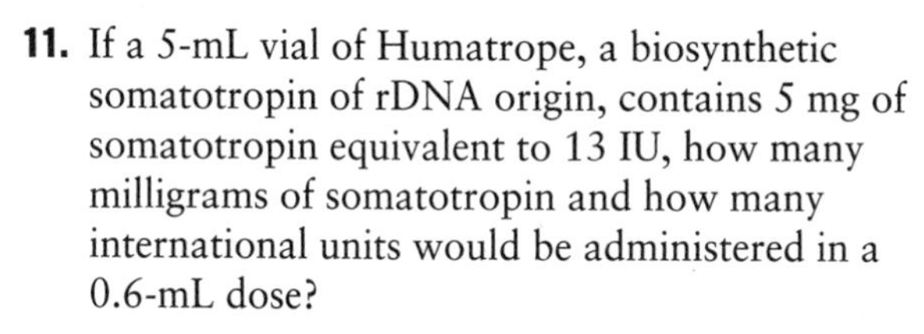

11. If a 5-mL vial of Humatrope, a biosynthetic somatotropin of rDNA origin, contains 5 mg of somatotropin equivalent to 13 IU, how many milligrams of somatotropin and how many international units would be administered in a 0.6-mL dose?

$$\frac{5 \text{ mg}}{5 \text{ mL}} \times 0.6 \text{ mL} = 0.6 \text{ mg}$$

$$\frac{13 \text{ IU}}{5 \text{ mL}} \times 0.6 \text{ mL} = 1.56 \text{ IU}$$

References

1. The United States Pharmacopeia. 24th Rev. and National Formulary, 19th Ed. Rockville, MD: The United States Pharmacopeial Convention, 2000.
2. Allen LV Jr. Formulations. International Journal of Pharmaceutical Compounding 1998;2:229.

5

DILUTION, CONCENTRATION, AND ALLIGATION

This chapter presents various types of calculations used to adjust the concentrations of preparations.

5.1 Dilution and Concentration

The strength of a pharmaceutical preparation is based on the quantity of the primary ingredient relative to the quantity of the preparation as a whole. A change in either of these two quantities results in a preparation of greater or lesser strength.

Definitions. In the present context, the term *dilution* means to diminish the strength of a preparation by the addition of solvent or vehicle. *Concentration* means to render a preparation to greater strength through a reduction in the relative quantity of solvent or vehicle.

Expression. The strengths of preparations subject to processes of dilution and concentration generally are expressed in terms of *percentage strength*.

Discussion. If a liquid preparation is diluted to twice its original quantity, its primary ingredient will be con-

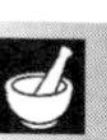

tained in twice as many parts of the whole, and therefore its strength will be reduced by one-half. Contrariwise, if a liquid preparation is concentrated by evaporation to one-half its original quantity, the primary ingredient will be contained in one-half as many parts of the whole, and its strength will be doubled. For example, if 50 mL of a solution containing 10 g of active ingredient (i.e., 20% weight-in-volume [w/v]) are diluted to 100 mL, the original volume is doubled, but the original strength is now reduced by one-half to 10% w/v (10 g/100 mL). If, by evaporation of the solvent, the volume of the solution is reduced to 25 mL or one-half the original quantity, the original strength is doubled to 40% w/v (10 g/25 mL). Similarly for solid preparations, such as ointments and powders, increasing the quantity of vehicle while maintaining the quantity of the active ingredient results in an inversely proportional reduction in strength.

Although problems in this section may be solved by other methods, use of the following equation is suggested.

$$(1^{st}\text{ quantity}) \times (1^{st}\text{ concentration}) = (2^{nd}\text{ quantity}) \times (2^{nd}\text{ concentration})$$

or

$$Q1 \times C1 = Q2 \times C2$$

Key Point. The percentage strength of a preparation is inversely proportional to a change in its total quantity. That is, an increase in total quantity results in a decrease in strength.

Pharmacy Applications. A pharmacist may use the necessary calculations and the needed processes of dilution or concentration to change the strength of a preparation to a strength desired.

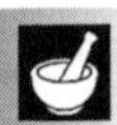

EXAMPLE PROBLEMS

1. If 500 mL of a 15% v/v solution is diluted to 1,500 mL, what is the resultant percentage strength?

Q1 (quantity) × C1 (concentration)
= Q2 (quantity) × C2 (concentration)

500 (mL) × 15 (%) = 1,500 (mL) × x (%)

1,500x = 7,500

x = 7,500 ÷ 1,500

x = 5% v/v

2. If a syrup containing 65% w/v of sucrose is evaporated to 85% of its volume, what percent of sucrose will it contain?

Note: any convenient volume of syrup may be selected, say 100 mL. Then, 85% × 100 mL = 85 mL (Q2)

Q1 × C1 = Q2 × C2

100 (mL) × 65 (%) = 85 (mL) × x (%)

85x = 6,500

x = 76.47% w/v

3. How many grams of 10% w/w ammonia solution can be made from 1,800 g of 28% w/w strong ammonia solution?

Q1 × C1 = Q2 × C2

1,800 (g) × 28 (%) = x (g) × 10 (%)

x = 5,040 g

4. If 1 gallon of a 30% w/v solution is evaporated so that the solution has a strength of 50% w/v, what is its volume in milliliters?

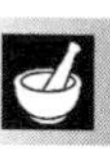

$Q1 \times C1 = Q2 \times C2$

$3{,}785\ (mL) \times 30\ (\%) = x\ (mL) \times 50\ (\%)$

$x = 2{,}271\ mL$

5. If 150 mL of a 17% w/v concentrate of benzalkonium chloride are diluted to 5 gallons, what will be the percentage strength of the dilution?

$5\ (gal) \times 3{,}785\ mL = 18{,}925\ mL$

$150\ (mL) \times 17\ (\%) = 18{,}925\ (mL) \times x\ (\%)$

$18{,}925x = 2{,}550$

$x = 0.13\%\ w/v$

6. How many grams of a 20% w/w benzocaine ointment and how many grams of ointment base should be used in preparing 5 lb of 2.5% benzocaine ointment?

$5\ (lb) \times 454\ g = 2{,}270\ g$

$2{,}270\ (g) \times 2.5\ (\%) = x\ (g) \times 20\ (\%)$

$20x = 5{,}675$

$x = 283.75\ g$ (20% ointment)

$2{,}270\ g - 283.75\ g = 1{,}986.25\ g$ (ointment base)

5.2 Stock Solutions

Stock solutions are used by pharmacists in compounding procedures.

Definition. A *stock solution* is a relatively concentrated solution of a medicinal or nonmedicinal substance used as the source of that substance to prepare a solution of lesser concentration.

Expression. Stock solutions may be expressed either in percentage strength or in ratio strength.

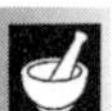

Discussion. Stock solutions may be obtained commercially or prepared by a pharmacist for use in compounding procedures. Depending on the physical nature of the primary agent, stock solutions may be calculated and prepared on a weight-in-volume (w/v) or volume-in-volume (v/v) basis. Because they are measured volumetrically, stock solutions provide a simple and convenient means of accurately obtaining an ingredient in the preparation of a liquid product.

EXAMPLE PROBLEMS

1. How many milliliters of a 1:400 w/v stock solution should be used to make 4 L of a 0.05% w/v solution?

4 L = 4,000 mL

1:400 w/v = 0.25% w/v

$Q1 \times C1 = Q2 \times C2$

$4{,}000 \text{ (mL)} \times 0.05 \text{ (\%)} = x \text{ (mL)} \times 0.25 \text{ (\%)}$

$x = 800 \text{ mL}$

2. How many milliliters of a 1% w/v stock solution of a certified red dye should be used in preparing 4,000 mL of a mouth wash that is to contain 1:20,000 w/v of the certified red dye as a coloring agent?

1:20,000 w/v = 0.005% w/v

$4{,}000 \text{ (mL)} \times 0.005 \text{ (\%)} = x \text{ (mL)} \times 1 \text{ (\%)}$

$x = 4{,}000 \times 0.005$

$x = 20 \text{ mL}$

3. How many milliliters of a 6.25% w/v solution of sodium hypochlorite should be used in preparing 5,000 mL of a 0.5% w/v solution of sodium hypochlorite for irrigation?

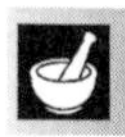

$5{,}000 \text{ (mL)} \times 0.5 \text{ (\%)} = x \text{ (mL)} \times 6.25 \text{ (\%)}$

$6.25x = 5{,}000 \times 0.5$

$x = 400 \text{ mL}$

4. How many milliliters of a 2% w/v stock solution of ephedrine sulfate should be used in compounding the following prescription?

℞ Ephedrine sulfate 0.25%

Rose water ad 30 mL

Sig. For the nose.

$30 \text{ (mL)} \times 0.25 \text{ (\%)} = x \text{ (mL)} \times 2 \text{ (\%)}$

$2x = 7.5$

$x = 3.75 \text{ mL}$

5. How many grams of silver nitrate should be used in preparing 50 mL of a solution such that 5 mL diluted to 500 mL will yield a 1:1,000 w/v solution?

1:1,000 w/v = 1 g of silver nitrate in 1,000 mL of solution or 0.1% w/v

$500 \text{ (mL)} \times 0.1 \text{ (\%)} = 5 \text{ (mL)} \times x \text{ (\%)}$

$5x = 50$

$x = 10 \text{ (\%)}$

Because the 5 mL is a 10% w/v solution, so is the 50 mL. Thus,

$50 \text{ mL} \times 10\% \text{ w/v} = 5 \text{ g}$

6. How many milliliters of a 17% w/v concentrate of benzalkonium chloride should be used in preparing 300 mL of a stock solution such that 15 mL diluted to 1 L will yield a 1:5,000 w/v solution?

1:5,000 w/v = 0.02% w/v

$1{,}000 \text{ (mL)} \times 0.02 \text{ (\%)} = 15 \text{ (mL)} \times x \text{ (\%)}$

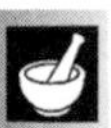

$15x = 20$

$x = 1.33\%$ w/v

Because the 15 mL is a 1.33% w/v solution, so is the 300 mL. Thus,

$300\ (\text{mL}) \times 1.33\ (\%) = 17\ (\%) \times x\ (\text{mL})$

$17x = 399$

$x = 23.47$ mL

5.3 Dilution of Acids

The strengths of concentrated and diluted acids are determined on a different basis, and thus the dilution of concentrated acids requires special calculations as described in this section.

Definition. In the present context, *dilution* is the reduction in strength of concentrated inorganic acids by admixture with water.

Expression. In the *United States Pharmacopeia* and *National Formulary,* the strengths of *concentrated* inorganic acids are expressed in percent weight-in-weight (w/w), and the strengths of *diluted* acids are expressed in percent weight-in-volume (w/v).[1]

Discussion. In diluting a concentrated acid, it is necessary to consider its strength and the desired strength of the diluted acid. Each concentrated acid has an individualized strength. For example, hydrochloric acid is 37% w/w HCl, nitric acid is 70% w/w HNO_3, and sulfuric acid is 97% w/w H_2SO_4. Counterpart diluted acids are 10% w/v unless stated otherwise. For safety in preventing acid spattering when diluting a concentrated acid, the acid is always added to the water.

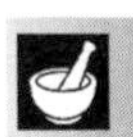

Key Point. Because concentrated acids are based on percent w/w and diluted acids are based on percent w/v, the use of specific gravity is required in certain calculations. For the definition and application of specific gravity, the reader may refer to Section 19.1 of this *Handbook*.

Pharmacy Applications. For the most part, inorganic acids are used in pharmacy in chemical/analytical procedures and only rarely in clinical application.

EXAMPLE PROBLEMS

1. How many milliliters of 37% w/w hydrochloric acid having a specific gravity of 1.20 are required to make 1,000 mL of diluted hydrochloric acid 10% w/v?

   Note: It is important to consider both the concentrated acid and the diluted acid on the same basis (i.e., w/w or w/v). Because the specific gravity of the concentrated acid is given, its w/w basis may be calculated on a w/v basis as follows:

   37% w/w = 37 g of HCl in each 100 g of concentrated acid

   100 g ÷ 1.20 (specific gravity) = 83.33 mL

   Thus, 37 g of HCl in 83.33 mL = 44.4% w/v

   $Q1 \times C1 = Q2 \times C2$

   $1{,}000\ (\text{mL}) \times 10\ (\%) = x\ (\text{mL}) \times 44.4\ (\%)$

   $44.4x = 10{,}000$

   $x = 225.23$ mL

2. How many milliliters of 85% w/w phosphoric acid having a specific gravity of 1.71 should be used in

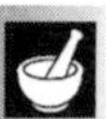

preparing 1 gallon of 0.25% w/v phosphoric acid solution to be used for bladder irrigation?

85% w/w = 85 g H_3PO_4 in each 100 g of concentrated acid

100 g ÷ 1.71 (specific gravity) = 58.48 mL

Thus, 85 g of H_3PO_4 in 58.48 mL = 145.35% w/v

3,785 (mL) × 0.25 (%) = x (mL) × 145.35 (%)

145.35x = 946.25

x = 6.51 mL

3. A pharmacist mixed 100 mL of 37% w/w concentrated hydrochloric acid (specific gravity, 1.20) with enough purified water to make 360 mL of diluted acid. Calculate the percentage strength (w/v) of the diluted acid.

100 mL × 1.20 (specific gravity)
= 120 g of concentrated acid

120 g × 37% w/w = 44.4 g HCl

$$\frac{44.4 \text{ g}}{360 \text{ mL}} \times 100 = 12.33\% \text{ w/v}$$

5.4 Triturations

A *trituration* is an example of a solid dilution.

Definition. *Triturations* are finely powdered dilutions of potent medicinal substances, with formerly official triturations containing 1 part of active constituent in 10 parts of mixture.

Expression. Triturations may be expressed either in percentage strength (for example, 10% w/w) or ratio strength (for example, 1:10 w/w).

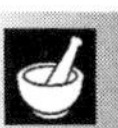

Discussion. Triturations were at one time an official type of pharmaceutical preparation. They were prepared by diluting 1 part by weight of the drug with 9 parts of finely powdered lactose for a total of 10 parts. These dilutions offered a convenient means of accurately obtaining small quantities of potent drugs for compounding purposes. Although no longer official, triturations exemplify a method for the calculation and use of dilutions of solid medicinal substances in compounding procedures.

Key Point. The term "trituration" as used in the present context should not be confused with the like term *trituration*, which is the pharmaceutical *process* of reducing substances to fine particles through grinding or milling.

Pharmacy Applications. A trituration may be prepared and used by a pharmacist to obtain a "weighable" quantity of a potent substance for use in compounding procedures. It should be recalled that the minimum quantity that should be weighed on a class A pharmacy balance is 120 mg (see Chapter 3). By weighing a trituration of the needed substance, rather than the pure substance itself, this requirement often may be met.

EXAMPLE PROBLEMS

1. How many grams of a 1:10 trituration are required to obtain 25 mg of drug?

10 g of trituration contain 1 g of drug

25 mg = 0.025 g

$$\frac{10\text{ g}}{1\text{ g}} \times 0.025\text{ g} = 0.25\text{ g}$$

2. How many milliliters of an injection prepared by dissolving 100 mg of a 1:10 trituration of

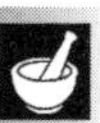

mechlorethamine hydrochloride in sufficient water for injection to prepare 10 mL of injection are required to obtain 5 mg of drug?

100 mg of 1:10 trituration = 10 mg of drug

10 mg of drug are present in 10 mL of injection

$$\frac{10 \text{ mL}}{10 \text{ mg}} \times 5 \text{ mg} = 5 \text{ mL}$$

3. How many milligrams of a 1:20 dilution of colchicine should be used by a manufacturing pharmacist in preparing 100 capsules for a clinical drug study if each capsule is to contain 0.5 mg of colchicine?

0.5 mg × 100 = 50 mg of colchicine needed

20 mg of dilution contain 1 mg of colchicine

$$\frac{20 \text{ mg}}{1 \text{ mg}} \times 50 \text{ mg} = 1{,}000 \text{ mg}$$

5.5 Alligation Medial

Alligation is an arithmetical method that is used for solving problems related to the mixing of preparations of different strengths. There are two types of alligation: *alligation medial*, discussed in this section, and *alligation alternate*, discussed in the next section.

Definition. *Alligation medial* is a method by which the weighted average of the strength, or other quantitative measure, of a mixture of two or more substances of known quantity and concentration is calculated.

Expression. The results of calculations by alligation medial may be expressed in percentage strength or in some other quantitative parameter.

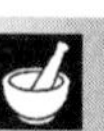

Discussion. Most often, alligation medial is used to determine the percentage strength of a mixture. By this method, the percentage strength of each component, expressed as a decimal fraction, is multiplied by its corresponding quantity, then the sum of the products is divided by the total quantity of the mixture, and the resultant decimal fraction is multiplied by 100 to give the percentage strength of the mixture. The quantities must be expressed in the same metric units, whether of weight or volume.

Alligation medial also may be used to determine the specific gravity of a mixture of liquids. As described in Section 19.1, specific gravity is calculated by:

$$\text{Specific gravity} = \frac{\text{Weight of the substance}}{\text{Weight of an equal volume of water}}$$

EXAMPLE PROBLEMS

1. What is the percentage strength (v/v) of alcohol in a mixture of 3,000 mL of 40% v/v alcohol, 1,000 mL of 60% v/v alcohol, and 1,000 mL of 70% v/v alcohol?

   40% × 3,000 mL = 1,200 mL
   60% × 1,000 mL = 600 mL
   70% × 1,000 mL = 700 mL
   Totals: 5,000 mL 2,500 mL
   2,500 (mL) ÷ 5,000 (mL) = 0.50 × 100 = 50% v/v

2. What is the percentage of zinc oxide in an ointment prepared by mixing 200 g of 10% w/w ointment, 50 g of 20% w/w ointment, and 100 g of 5% w/w ointment?

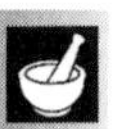

10% × 200 g = 20 g
20% × 50 g = 10 g
5% × 100 g = 5 g
Totals: 350 g 35 g
35 (g) ÷ 350 (g) = 0.10 × 100 = 10% w/w

3. What is the percent of alcohol in a mixture containing 500 mL of terpin hydrate elixir (40% v/v alcohol), 400 mL of theophylline sodium glycinate elixir (21% v/v alcohol), and sufficient simple syrup to make 1,000 mL?

Note: in problems in which a solvent or vehicle is present that contains no constituent on which the product's strength is based, it is calculated as zero percentage strength.

40% × 500 mL = 200 mL
21% × 400 mL = 84 mL
0% × 100 mL = 0 mL
Totals: 1,000 mL 284 mL
284 (mL) ÷ 1,000 (mL) = 0.284 × 100 = 28.4% v/v

4. Calculate the percentage of alcohol in the following prescription.

℞		
	Coal tar solution	80 mL (85% alcohol)
	Glycerin	160 mL
	Alcohol	500 mL (95% alcohol)
Boric acid solution ad		1,000 mL

85% × 80 mL = 68 mL
95% × 500 mL = 475 mL
Total: 543 mL

$543 \text{ (mL)} \div 1{,}000 \text{ (mL)} = 0.543 \times 100 = 54.3\% \text{ v/v}$

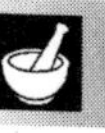

5. What is the specific gravity of a mixture of 1,000 mL of syrup with a specific gravity of 1.300, 400 mL of glycerin with a specific gravity of 1.250, and 1,000 mL of an elixir with a specific gravity of 0.950?

Note: specific gravity multiplied by volume in milliliters yields equivalent weight in grams.

$1.300 \times 1{,}000 \text{ (mL)} = 1{,}300 \text{ (g)}$

$1.250 \times 400 \text{ (mL)} = 500 \text{ (g)}$

$0.950 \times 1{,}000 \text{ (mL)} = 950 \text{ (g)}$

Totals: 2,400 (mL) 2,750 (g)

Specific gravity

$$= \frac{\text{Weight of the substance}}{\text{Weight of an equal volume of water}}$$

$$= \frac{2{,}750 \text{ (g)}}{2{,}400 \text{ (g)}} = 1.146$$

5.6 Alligation Alternate

Definition. *Alligation alternate* is an arithmetic method used to determine the quantities of two or more preparations of differing strengths to mix to achieve a final product of the desired quantity and strength.

Expression. The strengths of mixtures used in alligation alternate calculations are usually expressed in terms of percentage strength. The quantities produced by these calculations are usually expressed in parts, which can then be used to calculate actual amounts in grams or milliliters.

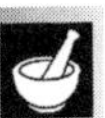

Discussion. The strength of a mixture of preparations lies somewhere between the strengths of its weaker and stronger components, but is always nearer to the strength of the component present in greater quantity. This weighted average can be found by a relatively simple method, as illustrated below.

Key Point. Although the problems presented in this section may be solved algebraically, as described in the textbook *Pharmaceutical Calculations*,[2] the method presented here works equally well.

Pharmacy Applications. Alligation alternate may be used by a pharmacist who wishes to determine the (1) relative amounts of preparations of different strengths to mix to achieve a product of the desired strength, (2) quantity of diluent to add to a preparation to reduce its strength, or (3) quantity of active constituent to add to a preparation to fortify its strength.

Diagrammatic Scheme for Alligation Alternate. The following scheme is used to determine the *relative proportion* of components to mix together to achieve a product of the desired percentage strength. The following problem demonstrates the application of this method.

> In what proportion should a 95% preparation and a 50% preparation be mixed to make a 70% preparation?

Note that the *difference* between the strength of the stronger component (95%) and the desired strength (70%) indicates the number of parts of the weaker to be used (i.e., 25 parts). The *difference* between the desired strength (70%) and the strength of the weaker component (50%) indicates the number of parts of the stronger

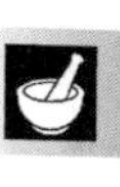

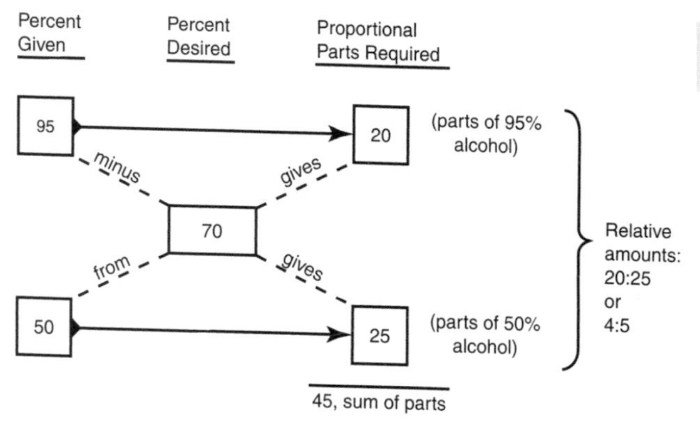

to be used (i.e., 20 parts). Thus, the proportion or ratio of the 95% and 50% preparations to use in making a 70% alcohol is 20:25, a *total* of 45 parts. The ratio may be reduced to 4:5, with a total of 9 parts. If, for example, 100 mL were to be prepared:

Each part would be equal to 11.11 mL [100 mL ÷ 9 (parts)], and therefore

44.44 mL of the 95% preparation [11.11 mL × 4 (parts)], and

55.55 mL of the 50% preparation [11.11 mL × 5 (parts)] would be needed.

The result can be shown to be correct by alligation medial:

$$0.95 \times 44.44 \text{ mL} = 42.218 \text{ mL}$$
$$0.50 \times \underline{55.55 \text{ mL}} = \underline{27.775 \text{ mL}}$$
$$\text{Totals: } 99.99 \text{ mL} \quad 69.993 \text{ mL}$$
$$69.993 \text{ (mL)} \div 99.99 \text{ (mL)} = 0.70 \times 100 = 70\% \text{ v/v}$$

EXAMPLE PROBLEMS

The layout of *alligation alternate,* used in the subsequent example problems, is a convenient simplification

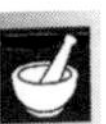

of the schematic diagram presented above. In the following problems, the strengths of inert bases are represented by 0% (meaning no active component) and of active components by 100%.

1. In what proportion should 20% benzocaine ointment be mixed with an ointment base to produce a 2.5% benzocaine ointment?

20%		2.5 parts of 20% ointment
	2.5%	
0%		17.5 parts of ointment base

Relative amounts = 2.5:17.5, or reduced = 1:7 (20% ointment : ointment base)

Proof of correctness of answer by alligation medial:

0.2×1 (part) $= 0.2$

$0 \times \underline{7}$ (parts) $= \underline{0}$

Totals: 8 0.2

$0.2 \div 8 = 0.025 \times 100 = 2.5\%$

2. A pharmacist wants to use two lots of ichthammol ointment containing 50% and 5% of ichthammol. In what proportion should they be mixed to prepare a 10% ichthammol ointment?

50%		5 parts of the 50% ointment
	10%	
5%		40 parts of the 5% ointment

Relative amounts = 5:40, or reduced = 1:8 (50% ointment : 5% ointment)

3. How many milliliters of 30% w/v dextrose solution and how many milliliters of 10% w/v dextrose solution are required to prepare 4,500 mL of a 15% w/v solution?

```
30% |        | 5 parts of the 30% solution
    | 15%    |
10% |        | 15 parts of the 10% solution
```

Relative amounts = 5:15, or reduced = 1:3 (30% solution : 10% solution)

Total parts = 4

Volume per part = 4,500 mL ÷ 4 (parts)

= 1,125 mL

Volume of the 30% solution = 1 (part) × 1,125 mL

= 1,125 mL

Volume of the 10% solution = 3 (parts) × 1,125 mL

= 3,375 mL

Or,

$$\frac{1 \text{ part } 30\% \text{ solution}}{4 \text{ parts total}} = \frac{x}{4{,}500 \text{ mL}}$$

x = 1,125 mL

$$\frac{3 \text{ parts } 10\% \text{ solution}}{4 \text{ parts total}} = \frac{x}{4{,}500 \text{ mL}}$$

x = 3,375 mL

4. How many milliliters each of 2% iodine tincture and 7% strong iodine tincture should be used in preparing 1 gallon of a tincture containing 3.5% iodine?

```
2% |        | 3.5 parts of the 2% tincture
   | 3.5%   |
7% |        | 1.5 parts of the 7% tincture
```

Relative amounts = 3.5:1.5, or reduced = 7:3 (2% tincture : 7% tincture)

Total parts = 10

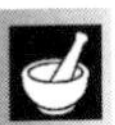

Volume per part = 3,785 mL ÷ 10 (parts)
= 378.5 mL

Volume of 2% tincture = 378.5 mL × 7 (parts)
= 2,649.5 mL

Volume of 7% tincture = 378.5 mL × 3 (parts)
= 1,135.5 mL

5. How many grams of 2.5% hydrocortisone cream should be mixed with 360 g of 0.25% cream to make a 1% hydrocortisone cream?

2.5%		0.75 part of the 2.5% cream
	1%	
0.25%		1.5 parts of the 0.25% cream

Relative amounts = 0.75:1.5, or reduced 1:2 (2.5% cream:0.25% cream)

$$\frac{\text{1 part 2.5\% cream}}{\text{2 parts 0.25\% cream}} = \frac{x}{\text{360 g}}$$

x = 180 g

6. How many grams of coal tar should be added to 3,200 g of 5% coal tar ointment to prepare an ointment containing 20% coal tar? Prove the answer by alligation medial.

100%		15 parts coal tar
	20%	
5%		80 parts of the 5% ointment

Relative amounts = 15:80, or reduced = 3:16 (coal tar:5% ointment)

$$\frac{\text{3 parts coal tar}}{\text{16 parts 5\% ointment}} = \frac{x}{\text{3,200 g}}$$

x = 600 g

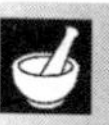

Proof of correctness of answer by alligation medial:

5% ×	3,200 g	= 160 g
100% ×	600 g	= 600 g
Totals:	3,800 g	760 g

760 g ÷ 3,800 g = 0.2 × 100 = 20% w/w

7. ℞ Hydrocortisone acetate ointment 10 g

0.25%

Sig. Apply to the eye.

How many grams of 2.5% ophthalmic hydrocortisone acetate ointment and how many grams of ophthalmic base (diluent) should be used in preparing the prescription?

2.5%		0.25
	0.25%	
0%		2.25

Total parts = 2.5

Grams per part = 10 g ÷ 2.5 = 4 g

Grams of 2.5% ointment = 0.25 (parts) × 4 g = 1 g

Grams of ointment base = 2.25 (parts) × 4 g = 9 g

8. ℞ Zinc oxide 1.5

Hydrophilic petrolatum 2.5

Purified water 5

Hydrophilic ointment ad 30

Sig. Apply to affected areas.

How many grams of zinc oxide should be added to the product to make an ointment containing 10% zinc oxide?

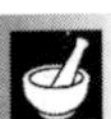

$$\frac{1.5 \text{ g}}{30 \text{ g}} \times 100$$

= 5% w/w (zinc oxide in the prescription)

5%		90
	10%	
100%		5

Relative amounts = 90:5, or reduced= 18:1 (prescription:zinc oxide)

$$\frac{18 \text{ parts prescription}}{1 \text{ part zinc oxide}} = \frac{30 \text{ g}}{\text{x}}$$

x = 1.667 g

Proof of answer:
Total zinc oxide = 1.5 g + 1.667 g = 3.167 g
Total weight of ointment = 30 g + 1.667 g
= 31.667 g

Percent of zinc oxide in ointment

$$= \frac{3.167}{31.667} \times 100 = 10\%$$

9. ℞[3] Cyclosporine 2%

Corn oil qs

Sig. Use as directed.

How many milliliters each of corn oil and a 10% solution of cyclosporine would be needed to prepare 30 mL of the prescription?

10%		2
	2%	
0%		8

Total parts = 10
Milliliters per part = 30 mL ÷ 10 (parts) = 3 mL

Milliliters of 10% cyclosporine

= 3 mL × 2 (parts) = 6 mL

Milliliters of corn oil = 3 mL × 8 parts = 24 mL

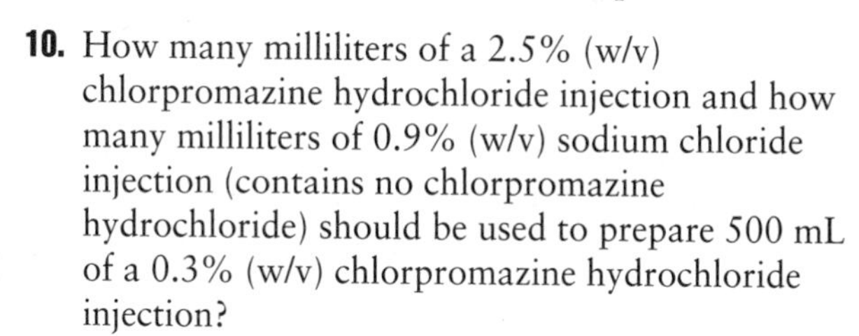

10. How many milliliters of a 2.5% (w/v) chlorpromazine hydrochloride injection and how many milliliters of 0.9% (w/v) sodium chloride injection (contains no chlorpromazine hydrochloride) should be used to prepare 500 mL of a 0.3% (w/v) chlorpromazine hydrochloride injection?

2.5%		0.3
	0.3%	
0%		2.2

Total parts = 2.5

Milliliters per part = 500 mL ÷ 2.5 = 200 mL

Milliliters of 2.5% chlorpromazine hydrochloride

= 200 mL × 0.3 (part) = 60 mL

Milliliters of 0.9% sodium chloride injection

= 200 mL × 2.2 (parts) = 440 mL

11. If an antibiotic injection contains 5% (w/v) of the drug, how many milliliters of diluent should be added to 5 mL of the injection to prepare a concentration of 5 mg of the antibiotic per milliliter?

5 mg = 0.005 g

$$\frac{0.005\ \text{g}}{1\ \text{mL}} \times 100 = 0.5\%$$

5%		0.5
	0.5%	
0%		4.5

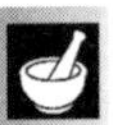

Relative amounts = 0.5:4.5, or reduced
= 1:9 (5% injection:diluent)

$$\frac{\text{1 part 5\% injection}}{\text{9 parts diluent}} = \frac{\text{5 mL}}{\text{x}}$$

x = 45 mL

12. How many milliliters of sterile water for injection should be added to a 1-mL vial containing 5 μg/mL of a drug to prepare a solution containing 1.5 μg/mL of the drug?

5 μg/mL		1.5
	1.5 μg/mL	
0 μg/mL		3.5

Relative amounts = 1.5:3.5, or reduced 3:7
(5 μg/mL vial:sterile water)

$$\frac{\text{3 parts 5 μg/mL}}{\text{7 parts sterile water}} = \frac{\text{1 mL}}{\text{x}}$$

x = 2.33 mL

References

1. The United States Pharmacopeia, 24th Rev. and National Formulary, 19th Ed. Rockville, MD: The United States Pharmacopeial Convention, 2000:2464–2465.
2. Ansel HC, Stoklosa MJ. Pharmaceutical Calculations. 11th Ed. Baltimore, MD: Lippincott Williams & Wilkins, 2001: 146–152.
3. Prince SJ. Calculations. International Journal of Pharmaceutical Compounding 2000;4:393.

6

REDUCING AND ENLARGING FORMULAS

Pharmacists may reduce or enlarge formulas for pharmaceutical preparations in the course of their professional practice or manufacturing activities. Official USP/NF formulas generally are based on the preparation of 1,000 mL or 1,000 g and may be reduced or enlarged as required. Industrial formulas for pharmaceutical products are scaled up from standard formulas to prepare production batches of hundreds of thousands of dosage units.

Definition. *Reducing or enlarging* a pharmaceutical formula is a process by which the total quantity is changed while the correct proportion of one ingredient to the other is maintained.

Expression. Components of formulas are expressed in units of weight or volume (usually metric) or in proportional parts.

Discussion. Each ingredient in a pharmaceutical formula relates proportionally to each of the other ingredients. If the quantity of one is changed, so must be the quantity of all others, such that their relationship one to the other is maintained. This ensures that no matter how much of the formula is prepared, it will have an identical composition. Most often, formulas are expressed in the metric

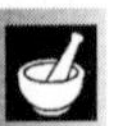

system. However, on occasion the relationship between ingredients may be expressed in the common systems of weights and measures or in proportional parts, such as "one part of glycerin for every two parts of water."

In reducing or enlarging a formula, only the numerical value of each ingredient is changed, and it does not matter whether the units of the individual ingredients are alike or different (e.g., grams or milliliters), as demonstrated in the example problems.

Pharmacy Applications. There are a number of instances in which a pharmacist may reduce or enlarge a formula. For example, on repeated calls for a compounded prescription for a specific patient, a pharmacist may prepare a larger quantity of the medication at one time for use in refilling the prescription. On the other hand, a pharmacist may reduce an established formula, such as one appearing in the USP/NF, to meet the one-time needs of a patient.

EXAMPLE PROBLEMS

1. From the following formula for calamine lotion, calculate the quantity of each ingredient required to make 240 mL.

Calamine	80 g
Zinc oxide	80 g
Glycerin	20 g
Bentonite magma	250 mL
Lime water ad	1,000 mL

Calamine: $\frac{80 \text{ g}}{1{,}000 \text{ mL}} \times 240 \text{ mL} = 19.2 \text{ g}$

Zinc oxide: $\frac{80 \text{ g}}{1{,}000 \text{ mL}} \times 240 \text{ mL} = 19.2 \text{ g}$

Glycerin: $\frac{20 \text{ mL}}{1{,}000 \text{ mL}} \times 240 \text{ mL} = 4.8 \text{ mL}$

Bentonite magma: $\frac{250 \text{ mL}}{1{,}000 \text{ mL}} \times 240 \text{ mL} = 60 \text{ mL}$

Lime water: to make 240 mL

2. From the following formula for 40 capsules, calculate the quantity of each ingredient required to make 16 capsules.

Belladonna extract	0.4 g
Ephedrine sulfate	0.64 g
Phenobarbital	0.8 g
Aspirin	12 g

Belladonna extract:

$$\frac{0.4 \text{ g}}{40 \text{ capsules}} \times 16 \text{ capsules} = 0.16 \text{ g}$$

Ephedrine sulfate:

$$\frac{0.64 \text{ g}}{40 \text{ capsules}} \times 16 \text{ capsules} = 0.256 \text{ g}$$

Phenobarbital:

$$\frac{0.8 \text{ g}}{40 \text{ capsules}} \times 16 \text{ capsules} = 0.32 \text{ g}$$

Aspirin:

$$\frac{12 \text{ g}}{40 \text{ capsules}} \times 16 \text{ capsules} = 4.8 \text{ g}$$

3. From the following formula, calculate the quantity of each ingredient required to make 1,000 g of the ointment.

Coal tar	5 parts
Zinc oxide	10 parts
Hydrophilic ointment	50 parts
Total number of parts	65

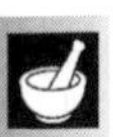

Coal tar: $\frac{5 \text{ parts}}{65 \text{ parts}} \times 1{,}000 \text{ g} = 76.923 \text{ g}$

Zinc oxide: $\frac{10 \text{ parts}}{65 \text{ parts}} \times 1{,}000 \text{ g} = 153.846 \text{ g}$

Hydrophilic ointment:

$$\frac{50 \text{ parts}}{65 \text{ parts}} \times 1{,}000 \text{ g} = 769.23 \text{ g}$$

Check: $76.923 + 153.846 + 769.23 \cong 1{,}000 \text{ g}$

4. From the following formula for a synthetic elastoviscous fluid for injection into the knee to treat osteoarthritis, calculate the quantities, in grams, of each of the first four ingredients needed to prepare five thousand 2-mL prefilled syringes.

Hylan polymers	80 mg
Sodium chloride	95 mg
Disodium hydrogen phosphate	1.5 mg
Sodium dihydrogen phosphate	0.4 mg
Water for injection ad	10 mL

$2 \text{ mL} \times 5{,}000 \text{ (syringes)} = 10{,}000 \text{ mL}$

Hylan polymers:

$$\frac{80 \text{ mg}}{10 \text{ mL}} \times 10{,}000 \text{ mL} = 80{,}000 \text{ mg} = 80 \text{ g}$$

Sodium chloride:

$$\frac{95 \text{ mg}}{10 \text{ mL}} \times 10{,}000 \text{ mL} = 95{,}000 \text{ mg} = 95 \text{ g}$$

Disodium hydrogen phosphate:

$$\frac{1.5 \text{ mg}}{10 \text{ mL}} \times 10{,}000 \text{ mL} = 1{,}500 \text{ mg} = 1.5 \text{ g}$$

Sodium dihydrogen phosphate:

$$\frac{0.4 \text{ mg}}{10 \text{ mL}} \times 10{,}000 \text{ mL} = 400 \text{ mg} = 0.4 \text{ g}$$

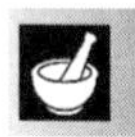

5. From the following formula for an oral electrolyte solution, calculate the amount of each ingredient required to prepare 480 mL of the solution.

Sodium	45 mEq
Potassium	20 mEq
Chloride	35 mEq
Citrate	30 mEq
Dextrose	25 g
Water ad	1,000 mL

Sodium: $\frac{45 \text{ mEq}}{1{,}000 \text{ mL}} \times 480 \text{ mL} = 21.6 \text{ mEq}$

Potassium: $\frac{20 \text{ mEq}}{1{,}000 \text{ mL}} \times 480 \text{ mL} = 9.6 \text{ mEq}$

Chloride: $\frac{35 \text{ mEq}}{1{,}000 \text{ mL}} \times 480 \text{ mL} = 16.8 \text{ mEq}$

Citrate: $\frac{30 \text{ mEq}}{1{,}000 \text{ mL}} \times 480 \text{ mL} = 14.4 \text{ mEq}$

Dextrose: $\frac{25 \text{ g}}{1{,}000 \text{ mL}} \times 480 \text{ mL} = 12 \text{ g}$

Water: ad 480 mL

6. A pediatric product is formulated to contain 100 mg of erythromycin ethylsuccinate in each dropperful (2.5 mL) of the product. How many grams of erythromycin ethylsuccinate would be required to prepare 5,000 bottles, each containing 50 mL of the preparation?

$$\frac{100 \text{ mg}}{2.5 \text{ mL}} \times \frac{1\text{g}}{1{,}000 \text{ mg}} \times \frac{50 \text{ mL}}{\text{bottle}} \times 5{,}000 \text{ bottles} = 10{,}000 \text{ g}$$

7

USE OF COMMERCIALLY PREPARED DOSAGE FORMS IN COMPOUNDING

In the extemporaneous compounding of prescriptions and medication orders, pharmacists often find that bulk supplies of certain pharmacologically active ingredients are not available and that commercially prepared dosage forms provide the only available source of the therapeutic agents needed.

7.1 Use of Tablets and Capsules in Compounding

Commercially prepared tablets and capsules commonly are used as the source of medicinal agents in extemporaneous compounding procedures. They are convenient, are quantitatively standardized, and often are available in various dosage strengths for compounding flexibility. Tablets and capsules may be used in the compounding of other solid dosage forms (e.g., powders) or in the preparation of semisolid or liquid forms. When only tablets or capsules of a specific therapeutic agent are commercially available, it is not uncommon for pharmacists to prepare counterpart liquid forms for children or adults who are unable to swallow solid dosage forms.

Discussion. Commercially prepared tablets and capsules vary in the complexity of their formulation. In compounding procedures, it is generally best to use dosage units that are of the simplest pharmaceutical form. For example, uncoated tablets are preferred over coated tablets. Controlled-release dosage forms are unsuitable for compounding. For convenience and economy, use of the fewest dosage units is preferred; for example, use of five 100-mg tablets is preferred over twenty-five 20-mg tablets.

When using tablets as the source of a therapeutic agent, the tablets are placed in a mortar and reduced to a powder. When capsules are used as the drug source, the capsule shells are opened, and their powdered contents are expelled. In either case, the exact number of dosage units is calculated, and the correct quantity of powder is used in the compounding procedure. It is important in certain calculations to account for the quantity of both the active and inactive ingredients in a solid dosage form. It should be recognized, for example, that a tablet labeled to contain 10 mg of a therapeutic agent may actually weigh substantially more because of the added ingredients.

EXAMPLE PROBLEMS

1. How many scored 100-mg allopurinol tablets should be used to prepare the following prescription?

℞	Allopurinol	65 mg/5 mL
	Cologel	40 mL
	Syrup ad	150 mL
	M. ft. susp.	
	Sig. As directed.	

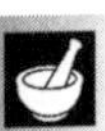

$$\frac{65 \text{ mg}}{5 \text{ mL}} \times 150 \text{ mL} = 1{,}950 \text{ mg}$$

$$1{,}950 \text{ mg} \times \frac{1 \text{ tablet}}{100 \text{ mg}} = 19.5 \text{ tablets}$$

2. How many 75-mg capsules of indomethacin should be used to prepare the following prescription?

℞		
	Indomethacin powder	1 %
	Carbopol 941 powder	2 %
	Purified water	10 %
	Alcohol ad	90 mL
	Sig. Use as directed.	

$$\frac{1 \text{ g}}{100 \text{ mL}} \times \frac{1{,}000 \text{ mg}}{1 \text{ g}} \times \frac{1 \text{ capsule}}{75 \text{ mg}} \times 90 \text{ mL} = 12 \text{ capsules}$$

3. How many 10-mg tablets of ketorolac tromethamine should be used to prepare the following prescription?

℞[1]		
	Ketorolac tromethamine	7.5 mg/5 mL
	Suspension vehicle ad	120 mL
	Sig. 1 tsp q6h	

$$\frac{7.5 \text{ mg}}{5 \text{ mL}} \times 120 \text{ mL} = 180 \text{ mg}$$

$$180 \text{ mg} \times \frac{1 \text{ tablet}}{10 \text{ mg}} = 18 \text{ tablets}$$

4. How many 0.75-mg tablets of estropipate should be used to prepare the following prescription?

℞		
	Estropipate	0.0125%
	Cream base ad	60 g
	Sig. Vaginal cream.	

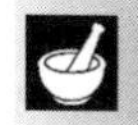

$$\frac{0.0125\text{ g}}{100\text{ g}} \times \frac{1{,}000\text{ mg}}{1\text{ g}} \times \frac{1\text{ tablet}}{0.75\text{ mg}} \times 60\text{ g} = 10\text{ tablets}$$

5. How many 20-mg tablets of enalapril, each weighing 120 mg, and how many grams of lactose should be used to prepare the following prescription?

℞	Enalapril	7.5 mg
	Lactose ad	200 mg
	DTD caps #40	
	Sig. Take one capsule each morning.	

7.5 mg/capsule × 40 capsules
= 300 mg (enalapril needed to fill the ℞)

$$300\text{ mg} \times \frac{1\text{ tablet}}{20\text{ mg}} = 15\text{ tablets needed to fill the ℞}$$

15 tablets × 120 mg (weight of 1 tablet)
= 1,800 mg (weight of 15 tablets)

200 mg (weight of contents of 1 capsule for ℞)
× 40 (capsules) = 8,000 mg
(weight of contents of 40 capsules)

8,000 − 1,800 mg = 6,200 mg
= 6.2 g of lactose needed to fill ℞

6. A starting pediatric dose of Dilantin sodium (phenytoin sodium) is 6 mg/kg/day, administered in three equally divided doses. Using tablets containing 50 mg of phenytoin sodium, a pharmacist wants to prepare a suspension such that each 1 mL, to be delivered by calibrated dropper, contains a single dose for a 44-lb child. How many tablets should be used to prepare 30 mL of the suspension?

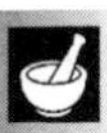

$$\frac{6 \text{ mg}}{1 \text{ kg/day}} \times \frac{1 \text{ kg}}{2.2 \text{ lb}} \times 44 \text{ lb} = 120 \text{ mg/day}$$

$$120 \text{ mg} \div 3 \text{ (doses/day)} = 40 \text{ mg/dose}$$

$$\frac{40 \text{ mg}}{1 \text{ mL}} \times 30 \text{ mL}$$

$$= 1{,}200 \text{ (phenytoin sodium needed in ℞)}$$

$$1{,}200 \text{ mg} \times \frac{1 \text{ tablet}}{50 \text{ mg}} = 24 \text{ tablets}$$

7.2 Use of Injections in Compounding

Small-volume injections may be injected directly into patients or added to large-volume parenterals for intravenous infusion, as discussed in Chapter 14. They also may be used as the source of therapeutic agents in compounding procedures.

Expressions. The concentrations of therapeutic agents in injections generally are expressed in *percentage strength* or in terms of *quantity per unit volume* (e.g., mg/mL, units/mL, mEq/mL).

Discussion. Because injections are liquids, they are especially useful in preparing other liquid dosage forms such as oral solutions and suspensions and some semisolid preparations that can adequately absorb the added liquid. When used, the calculated volume of injection should be accurately withdrawn from an ampul or vial using a calibrated syringe.

EXAMPLE PROBLEMS

1. The following is a formula for a diazepam rectal gel.[2] How many 10-mL vials of an injection

containing 5 mg/mL of diazepam would be needed to prepare the formula?

Diazepam	100 mg
Methylcellulose (1,500 cps)	2.5 g
Methylparaben	100 mg
Glycerin	5 g
Purified water ad	100 mL

$$\frac{5 \text{ mg}}{1 \text{ mL}} \times 10 \text{ mL} = 50 \text{ mg/vial}$$

$$100 \text{ mg} \times \frac{1 \text{ vial}}{50 \text{ mg}} = 2 \text{ vials}$$

2. How many milliliters of an injection containing 40 mg of a drug per milliliter would provide the amount of the drug needed to prepare 120 mL of a 0.2% suspension?

$$\frac{0.2 \text{ g}}{100 \text{ mL}} \times \frac{1{,}000 \text{ mg}}{1 \text{ g}} \times \frac{1 \text{ mL}}{40 \text{ mg}} \times 120 \text{ mL} = 6 \text{ mL}$$

3. How many milliliters of an injection containing 40 mg of triamcinolone per milliliter may be used to prepare the following prescription?

℞		
	Triamcinolone	0.05%
	Ointment base ad	60 g

$$\frac{0.05 \text{ g}}{100 \text{ g}} \times \frac{1{,}000 \text{ mg}}{1 \text{ g}} \times \frac{1 \text{ mL}}{40 \text{ mg}} \times 60 \text{ g} = 0.75 \text{ mL}$$

References

1. Prince SJ. Calculations. International Journal of Pharmaceutical Compounding 1998;2:164.
2. Allen LV Jr. Diazepam dosed as a rectal gel. U S Pharmacist 2000;25:98.

8 MISCELLANEOUS COMPOUNDING CALCULATIONS

The pharmacist may compound many different dosage forms. However, capsules and suppositories present unique challenges, which are discussed in this chapter.

8.1 Capsule Filling

Properly prepared capsules should be completely filled, with no air pockets within the capsule shell. Choosing an appropriate-sized capsule and adding the required amount of a diluent if needed can accomplish this. Different powders will pack into a capsule shell to varying degrees. Some powders will pack tightly, and a relatively large quantity of the powder can be packed into the capsule shell; on the other hand, some powders will pack loosely, and only a small quantity can be packed into the capsule shell.

The example prescription used throughout this section is as follows:

℞ Drug A 20 mg
Drug B 55 mg
M. ft. caps #20

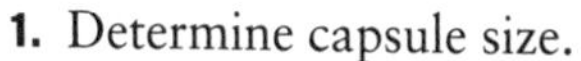

1. Determine capsule size.
   Capsule shells for human use are available in sizes 000, 00, 0, 1, 2, 3, 4, and 5, with 000 being the largest and 5 being the smallest size (Fig. 8-1). The following table can be used to determine the capsule size needed for a specified amount of powder.

Capsule Size	Approximate Volume[1]	Approximate Amount of Powder[2]
000	1.4 mL	0.43–1.8 g
00	0.95 mL	0.39–1.3 g
0	0.68 mL	325–900 mg
1	0.5 mL	227–650 mg
2	0.37 mL	200–520 mg
3	0.3 mL	120–390 mg
4	0.21 mL	100–260 mg
5	0.13 mL	65–130 mg

   In many cases, the amount of drug in each capsule will not be the determining factor in choosing the capsule size because of the small doses of most drugs. When considering patient convenience, capsule sizes of 0 to 3 are appropriate because they are small enough to be easily swallowed but not so small that the patient will have difficulty handling them.
2. Calculate diluent requirement.
   For the capsule to be completely filled, a diluent must be added in most cases. It is important to determine the volume of diluent powder that is equivalent to the required volume of drug or excipient powder to prepare the capsules correctly.

A. Weigh a capsule filled with each drug and diluent.
When weighing capsules, only the contents of the capsule should be weighed, and not the capsule shell. Using the example prescription, assume the following:

Size 1 capsule full of Drug A weighs 620 mg
Size 1 capsule full of Drug B weighs 470 mg
Size 1 capsule full of diluent weighs 330 mg

B. Calculate diluent displacement for each ingredient.
The diluent displacement is calculated by setting up a ratio of the weights of the individual ingredients to the weight of the diluent compared with the weight of the drug in each prescribed capsule as follows:

$$\frac{620 \text{ mg}}{330 \text{ mg}} = \frac{20 \text{ mg}}{x} \qquad x = 10.65 \text{ mg}$$

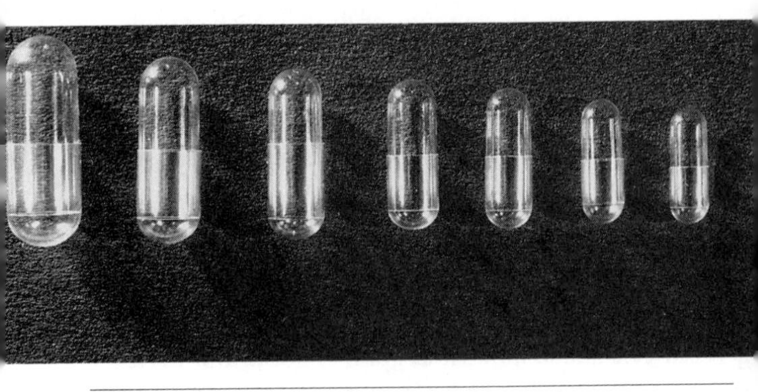

FIGURE 8-1. Actual sizes of hard gelatin capsules. From left to right, sizes 000, 00, 0, 1, 2, 3, 4, and 5. (Reprinted with permission from Ansel HC, Allen LV, Popovich NG. Pharmaceutical Dosage Forms and Drug Delivery Systems. 7th Ed. Baltimore, MD: Lippincott Williams & Wilkins, 1999:185.)

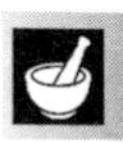

$$\frac{470 \text{ mg}}{330 \text{ mg}} = \frac{55 \text{ mg}}{x} \qquad x = 38.62 \text{ mg}$$

Total = 10.65 mg + 38.62 mg = 49.27 mg

20 mg of Drug A displaces 10.65 mg of diluent, and 55 mg of Drug B displaces 38.62 mg of diluent; therefore, 49.27 mg of total diluent is displaced.

C. Calculate amount of diluent required per capsule. The amount of diluent required per capsule is the diluent displacement subtracted from the weight of the capsule full of diluent.

330 mg − 49.27 mg
= 280.73 mg of diluent per capsule

3. Determine the total weight of each capsule.
To determine the weight of each capsule, the weights of each ingredient per capsule are simply added. It is important not to confuse the diluent displacements with the actual weight of the ingredients. In the example prescription, each capsule should contain 20 mg of Drug A and 55 mg of Drug B, not 10.65 mg and 38.62 mg, respectively.

20 mg + 55 mg + 280.73 mg
= 355.73 mg of powder mixture in each capsule

4. Calculate total amount of each ingredient needed to fill the prescription.
Multiply the quantity of each ingredient by the number of capsules to be prepared. It may be necessary to calculate for extra capsules to allow for some waste in the filling process. Usually calculating for two extra capsules will allow adequate powder to account for waste. However, this may not be feasible if the prescription includes a controlled sub-

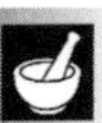

stance that must be inventoried. The calculated amounts of each ingredient are then weighed and mixed uniformly.

$$\text{Drug A: } \frac{20 \text{ mg}}{1 \text{ capsule}} \times 22 \text{ capsules} = 440 \text{ mg}$$

$$\text{Drug B: } \frac{55 \text{ mg}}{1 \text{ capsule}} \times 22 \text{ capsules} \times \frac{1 \text{ g}}{1{,}000 \text{ mg}} = 1.21 \text{ g}$$

$$\text{Diluent: } \frac{280.73 \text{ mg}}{1 \text{ capsule}} \times 22 \text{ capsules} \times \frac{1 \text{ g}}{1{,}000 \text{ mg}} = 6.18 \text{ g}$$

5. Fill and weigh each capsule.
   Each capsule shell is packed with the powder mixture and weighed to ensure that the prescribed amount of drug is contained in each capsule.

EXAMPLE PROBLEM

A pharmacist needs to prepare 50 capsules, each containing 4 mg of estriol and 1 mg of estradiol. A size 3 capsule is chosen for this prescription, and separate capsules are filled with each drug and lactose. The weights of the contents of each capsule are as follows: estriol = 250 mg, estradiol = 190 mg, and lactose = 320 mg.[3]

A. How much of each ingredient will be needed to prepare this prescription? (Do not account for extra capsules.)

   Lactose displacement:

   Estriol:

$$\frac{250 \text{ mg}}{320 \text{ mg}} = \frac{4 \text{ mg}}{x} \qquad x = 5.12 \text{ mg lactose}$$

Estradiol:

$$\frac{190 \text{ mg}}{320 \text{ mg}} = \frac{1 \text{ mg}}{x} \qquad x = 1.68 \text{ mg lactose}$$

Total amount of lactose displaced:

$$5.12 \text{ mg} + 1.68 \text{ mg} = 6.8 \text{ mg}$$

Amount of lactose per capsule:

$$320 \text{ mg} - 6.8 \text{ mg} = 313.2 \text{ mg}$$

$$\frac{4 \text{ mg estriol}}{1 \text{ capsule}} \times 50 \text{ capsules} = 200 \text{ mg estriol}$$

$$\frac{1 \text{ mg estradiol}}{1 \text{ capsule}} \times 50 \text{ capsules} = 50 \text{ mg estradiol}$$

$$\frac{313.2 \text{ mg lactose}}{1 \text{ capsule}} \times 50 \text{ capsules} \times \frac{1 \text{ g}}{1{,}000 \text{ mg}} = 15.66 \text{ g lactose}$$

B. How much should each capsule weigh?

$$4 \text{ mg} + 1 \text{ mg} + 313.2 \text{ mg} = 318.2 \text{ mg}$$

8.2 Suppository Molding

Before suppositories can be accurately prepared by molding, the mold must be calibrated by determining the volume of the suppository cavities. This can be accomplished by preparing suppositories containing no medication from a base material with a known density. The average weight of the suppositories is obtained, and the volume of each suppository is calculated by dividing this weight by the density of the base used. For example, an uncalibrated suppository mold is used to prepare 10 suppositories from cocoa butter alone (density of cocoa butter is 0.86 g/mL). After the suppositories are allowed to cool and harden, they are removed from the mold and

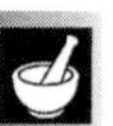

weighed at 18.8 g. The calibrated volume of this mold would then be:

$$\frac{18.8 \text{ g}}{10 \text{ suppositories}} = 1.88 \text{ g/suppository}$$

$$\frac{1.88 \text{ g}}{1 \text{ suppository}} \times \frac{1 \text{ mL}}{0.86 \text{ g}} = 2.19 \text{ mL/suppository}$$

To ensure that the correct amount of drug is contained in each suppository, the volume occupied by the drug and amount of suppository base displaced must be considered. However, if the quantity of active drug is less than 100 mg in a 2-g suppository, the volume of drug is probably insignificant and may not be taken into account. There are several methods for determination of dose replacement for suppositories: dosage replacement factor, density factor, and occupied volume.[4] These methods, however, are beyond the scope of this *Handbook*, and the reader should refer to Ansel et al[4] for a detailed discussion of these methods. The method presented below is a practical approach that can be used for any suppository formula and does not require the use of specific equations or information.

The example prescription used throughout this section is as follows:

℞ Drug C 350 mg
M. ft. supp #12

1. Weigh the active ingredient for the preparation of a single suppository.
   Accurately weigh 350 mg of Drug C.
2. Dissolve or mix it with a portion of melted base insufficient to fill one cavity of the mold.
   Accurately weigh 1 g of suppository base, melt the base in a small glass beaker, and add 350 mg of Drug C.

3. Add the mixture to a cavity.
4. Add additional melted base to the cavity to fill it completely.
5. Allow the suppository to congeal and harden.
6. Remove the suppository from the mold and weigh it. *The suppository containing 350 mg of Drug C is found to weigh 1.95 g.*
7. The weight of drug subtracted from the weight of the suppository gives the amount of base needed.

$$1.95\text{ g} - \left(350\text{ mg} \times \frac{1\text{ g}}{1{,}000\text{ mg}}\right) = 1.6\text{ g of base per suppository}$$

The above process and calculations should be repeated at least twice and an average obtained to avoid any errors in weighing or measuring. To complete the prescription, the total amount of drug and base should be calculated. Enough material for two extra suppositories should be included to allow for overfill of the mold.

$$\frac{350\text{ mg}}{1\text{ suppository}} \times \frac{1\text{ g}}{1{,}000\text{ mg}} \times 14\text{ suppositories} = 4.9\text{ g of Drug C needed}$$

$$\frac{1.6\text{ g}}{1\text{ suppository}} \times 14\text{ suppositories} = 22.4\text{ g of base needed}$$

EXAMPLE PROBLEMS

1. A pharmacist prepares six suppositories from a polyethylene glycol base with a density of 1.18 g/mL. The total weight of the suppositories is 13.81 g. What is the calibrated volume of the mold?

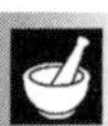

$$\frac{13.81\text{ g}}{6\text{ suppositories}} = 2.3\text{ g/suppository}$$

$$\frac{2.3\text{ g}}{1\text{ suppository}} \times \frac{1\text{ mL}}{1.18\text{ g}} = 1.95\text{ mL/suppository}$$

2.[5] ℞ Fluconazole 200 mg
Polyethylene glycol (PEG) base q.s.
M. ft. supp #20

Fill in the blanks for the method of preparation:

A. Weigh _____ of fluconazole.

200 mg

B. Mix the fluconazole with 1.1 g of the PEG base.

C. Melt the mixture and pour into a cavity in the suppository mold.

D. Melt approximately 1 g of the PEG base alone and add enough to the cavity to completely fill it.

E. Allow the suppository to cool and weigh it. (*You find that it weighs 2.4 g.*)

F. Weigh ________ of fluconazole and ________ of PEG base to fill the prescription. (Do not calculate for extra suppositories.)

$$\frac{200\text{ mg fluconazole}}{1\text{ suppository}} \times 20\text{ suppositories} \times \frac{1\text{ g}}{1{,}000\text{ mg}} = 4\text{ g of fluconazole}$$

$$2.4\text{ g} - \left(200\text{ mg} \times \frac{1\text{ g}}{1{,}000\text{ mg}}\right) = 2.2\text{ g of base per suppository}$$

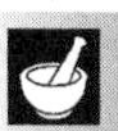

$$\frac{2.2 \text{ g base}}{1 \text{ suppository}} \times 20 \text{ suppositories} = 44 \text{ g of base}$$

References

1. Ansel HC, Allen LV, Popovich NG. Pharmaceutical Dosage Forms and Drug Delivery Systems. 7th Ed. Baltimore, MD: Lippincott Williams & Wilkins, 1999:185.
2. Product: Empty Gelatin Capsules. Indianapolis, IN: Eli Lilly and Company.
3. Prince SJ. Calculations. International Journal of Pharmaceutical Compounding 1999:3:408.
4. Ansel HC, Allen LV, Popovich NG. Pharmaceutical Dosage Forms and Drug Delivery Systems. 7th Ed. Baltimore, MD: Lippincott Williams & Wilkins, 1999:288–290.
5. Allen LV. The Art, Science, and Technology of Pharmaceutical Compounding. Washington, DC: American Pharmaceutical Association, 1997:140.

9

ISOTONIC SOLUTIONS

Aqueous pharmaceutical preparations intended for use in the bloodstream, eye, nose, or bowel generally are prepared to have the desired *tone* or *tonicity* with respect to the biologic fluids they encounter.

By physical law, when two solutions are placed on either side of a semipermeable membrane, solvent passes through the membrane from the more dilute solution toward the more concentrated solution to equalize the concentrations. This process is known as *osmosis,* and the pressure responsible for the movement of the solvent is termed *osmotic pressure*.

The effective osmotic pressure of a solution varies with the solute present. If the solute is a nonelectrolyte, its solution contains only unionized molecules and the osmotic pressure is determined solely by the concentration of the solute. If the solute is an electrolyte, its solution will contain ions and the osmotic pressure is determined not only by the solute's concentration but also by its degree of dissociation. Solutes that dissociate have a relatively greater number of particles in solution and exert a greater osmotic pressure than undissociated molecules.

Two solutions that have the same osmotic pressure are termed *isosmotic*. Many solutions intended to be mixed with body fluids are designed to have the same osmotic pressure for greater comfort, efficacy, and safety. A solution having the same osmotic pressure as a partic-

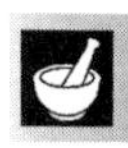

ular body fluid is said to be *isotonic* (meaning of equal tone) with that specific body fluid.

Solutions of lesser osmotic pressure than that of a body fluid are termed *hypotonic,* whereas those having a greater osmotic pressure are termed *hypertonic.* A hypotonic solution tends to lose solvent by osmosis through a semipermeable biologic membrane (such as that of a red blood cell), whereas a hypertonic solution tends to draw fluid and expand the volume of the extracellular liquid. A hypertonic laxative, for example, draws fluid from the surrounding tissues, thereby expanding the volume of liquid within the bowel.

9.1 The Dissociation Factor of an Electrolyte

Osmotic pressure and therefore a solution's tonicity are affected by the number of particles in solution. Substances that dissociate have greater tonic effect than substances that do not dissociate. Thus, the greater the dissociation, the greater the osmotic pressure and tonic effect.

Definition. The dissociation factor is a measure of the number of particles that effectively results when a substance is placed in aqueous solution.

Expression. The dissociation factor is symbolized by the letter i.

Discussion. Nonelectrolytes and substances subject to only slight dissociation are assigned an i factor of 1.0. Sodium chloride in weak solutions is about 80% dissociated, and therefore each 100 molecules yields 180 particles, or 1.8 times as many as are yielded by 100 molecules of a nonelectrolyte. Thus, sodium chloride is

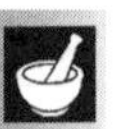

assigned an i factor of 1.8. As shown by the example problems below, if the dissociation of a solute is known, its corresponding i factor may be calculated.

The i factors for many medicinal substances vary depending on the concentration in solution. Dissociation factors may be determined experimentally or approximations made based on comparison with the known i factors of similar compounds in weak solutions. Thus, lacking better information, the following i factors may be assumed:

Nonelectrolytes and substances of slight dissociation: $i = 1.0$
Substances that dissociate into two ions: $i = 1.8$
Substances that dissociate into three ions: $i = 2.6$
Substances that dissociate into four ions: $i = 3.4$
Substances that dissociate into five ions: $i = 4.2$

Pharmacy Application. The i factor of a substance may be used to determine its *sodium chloride equivalent* (see Section 9.2), and thus the quantity needed to prepare a pharmaceutical preparation of the desired tonicity.

EXAMPLE PROBLEMS

1. Zinc sulfate is a two-ion electrolyte, dissociating 40% in weak solutions. Calculate its dissociation factor.

On the basis of 40% dissociation, 100 particles of zinc sulfate ($ZnSO_4$) yield:

40 zinc ions
40 sulfate ions
60 undissociated particles
140 total particles

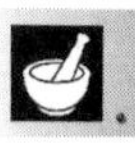

Because 140 particles represent 1.4 times as many particles as were present before dissociation, the dissociation factor is 1.4.

2. Zinc chloride ($ZnCl_2$) is a three-ion electrolyte, dissociating 80% in weak solutions. Calculate its dissociation factor.

   On the basis of 80% dissociation, 100 particles of zinc chloride will yield:

   80 zinc ions
   160 chloride ions
   20 undissociated particles
   260 total particles

   Because 260 particles represent 2.6 times as many particles as were present before dissociation, the dissociation factor is 2.6.

9.2 Sodium Chloride Equivalents

Definition. The relative quantity of a substance equal in tonic effect to sodium chloride is termed its *sodium chloride equivalent.*

Expression. Sodium chloride equivalents (*E* values) are expressed in decimal fractions.

Discussion. A 0.9% sodium chloride solution is considered to be isotonic with body fluids. When hypotonic, isotonic, or hypertonic solutions are to be prepared using agents other than sodium chloride, it is important to be able to determine the tonic effect of that other substance in terms of sodium chloride

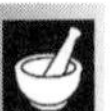

equivalence. As the standard, sodium chloride is assigned a *sodium chloride equivalent* of 1.0. All other agents are calculated as a decimal fraction of this standard. For example, an agent with a sodium chloride equivalent of 0.8 contributes eight-tenths or 80% as much toward tonicity as an equivalent quantity of sodium chloride.

Sodium chloride equivalents for a number of agents may be determined experimentally, or they may be calculated by the following formula:

$$\frac{\text{Molecular weight of sodium chloride}}{i \text{ factor of sodium chloride}} \times \frac{i \text{ factor of the substance}}{\text{Molecular weight of the substance}} = \text{Sodium chloride equivalent}$$

So, for example, the sodium chloride equivalent for zinc chloride may be calculated as follows:

Sodium chloride:

Molecular weight = 58.5

i factor = 1.8 (NaCl, two ions)

Zinc chloride:

Molecular weight = 136

i factor = 2.6 ($ZnCl_2$, three ions)

$$\frac{58.5}{1.8} \times \frac{2.6}{136} = 0.62$$

Pharmacy Applications. As described in Section 9.3, sodium chloride equivalents are used in the calculations needed to prepare pharmaceutical solutions of the desired tonicity.

EXAMPLE PROBLEMS

1. Calculate the sodium chloride equivalent for glycerin, a nonelectrolyte with a molecular weight of 92.

   i factor for sodium chloride = 1.8

   i factor for glycerin = 1.0

   $$\frac{58.5}{1.8} \times \frac{1.0}{92} = 0.35$$

2. Calculate the sodium chloride equivalent for timolol maleate, which dissociates into two ions and has a molecular weight of 432.

   i factor for sodium chloride = 1.8

   i factor for timolol maleate = 1.8

   $$\frac{58.5}{1.8} \times \frac{1.8}{432} = 0.14$$

3. Calculate the sodium chloride equivalent for fluorescein sodium, which dissociates into three ions and has a molecular weight of 376.

   i factor for sodium chloride = 1.8

   i factor for fluorescein sodium = 2.6

   $$\frac{58.5}{1.8} \times \frac{2.6}{367} = 0.22$$

9.3 Preparation of Isotonic Solutions

Definition. An *isotonic solution* is a solution that has the same tone as the biologic fluid with which it is intended to be mixed, generally considered the equivalent of 0.9% sodium chloride.

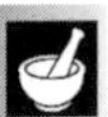

Expression. Isotonic solutions may be expressed with respect to their relation to a specific biologic fluid, as *isotonic with blood* or *isotonic with tears.*

Discussion. As stated above, an isotonic solution is one that contains the equivalent of 0.9% sodium chloride, or 0.9 g of sodium chloride per 100 mL of solution. When substances other than sodium chloride are used, an isotonic solution may still be calculated by applying the sodium chloride equivalent(s) of the other substance(s). For example, if a substance with a sodium chloride equivalent of 0.5 is used, 1.8 g (0.9 g ÷ 0.5) of that agent per 100 mL of solution would provide a tonic effect equivalent to that of 0.9% sodium chloride. It is recalled that a sodium chloride equivalent of 0.5 means that a substance is one-half as capable of providing tonicity as sodium chloride and thus, in the example, twice as much of the agent as sodium chloride is required. On the same basis, a substance with an *E* value of 0.2 would require 4.5 g (0.9 g ÷ 0.2) to prepare 100 mL of an isotonic solution, a substance with an *E* value of 0.6 would require 1.5 g (0.9 g ÷ 0.6), a substance with an *E* value of 0.8 would require 1.125 g (0.9 g ÷ 0.8), and so forth. In these examples, 4.5 g, 1.5 g, and 1.125 g of each of these substances would have a tonic effect equivalent to that of 0.9 g of sodium chloride.

As a corollary calculation, if, for example, 4.5 g of a substance is used to prepare 100 mL of an isotonic solution, the quantity of that substance is the equivalent of 0.9 g of sodium chloride in tonic effect and its sodium chloride equivalent may be calculated as 0.2 (0.9 g ÷ 4.5 g).

In some pharmaceutical preparations, sodium chloride and/or other agents may be present that contribute to the tonicity of a solution, and the contribution of each may be calculated. For example, if 30 mL of an

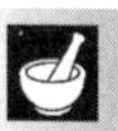

ophthalmic solution is to be prepared to be isotonic with tears, the equivalent of 0.9% sodium chloride or 0.27 g (30 mL × 0.9% w/v) of sodium chloride would be required. If the solution is prepared to contain, say, 1% atropine sulfate with a sodium chloride equivalent of 0.12, 0.3 g of atropine sulfate would be used (30 mL × 1% = 0.3 g), which would be equivalent in tonic effect to 0.036 g of sodium chloride (0.3 g × 0.12 = 0.036 g). By subtraction, 0.234 g of sodium chloride would be needed to render the solution isotonic (0.27 g − 0.036 g = 0.234 g).

The general procedure for the calculation of isotonic solutions using sodium chloride equivalents is as follows:

Step 1. Calculate the quantity, in grams, of sodium chloride alone that would be required to prepare an isotonic solution (0.9% w/v) of the volume specified in the prescription or formula.

Step 2. Calculate the tonic effect represented by each ingredient in a prescription or formula by multiplying each quantity, in grams, by its sodium chloride equivalent.

Step 3. Subtract the amount of sodium chloride represented by the ingredients from the amount of sodium chloride alone that would be required. The answer represents the quantity of sodium chloride to be added to render the solution isotonic.

Step 4. If an agent other than sodium chloride (e.g., boric acid, dextrose, etc.) is to be used to make the solution isotonic, divide the quantity of sodium chloride required in Step 3 by the sodium chloride equivalent of the agent to be used.

Key Point. If the number of grams of a substance included in a prescription or formula is multiplied by its

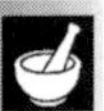

sodium chloride equivalent, its tonic effect equivalent to that amount of sodium chloride is determined.

Pharmacy Applications. The calculations in this chapter may be applied in the determination of solutions that are hypotonic, isotonic, or hypertonic.

EXAMPLE PROBLEMS

Note: the sodium chloride equivalents (*E* values) used in solving the following and other problems may be found in Appendix B.

1. How many grams of sodium chloride should be used in compounding the following prescription?

℞		
	Pilocarpine nitrate	0.3 g
	Sodium chloride	q.s.
	Purified water ad	30 mL
	Make isoton. sol.	
	Sig. For the eye.	

Step 1. 30 mL × 0.9% w/v = 0.27 g of sodium chloride or its equivalent needed to prepare 30 mL of an isotonic solution.

Step 2. 0.3 g × 0.23 (*E* value) = 0.069 g of sodium chloride equivalence represented by the pilocarpine nitrate.

Step 3. 0.27 g − 0.069 g = 0.201 g of sodium chloride required.

2. How many grams of boric acid should be used in compounding the following prescription?

℞		
	Phenacaine hydrochloride	1%
	Chlorobutanol	0.5%
	Boric acid	q.s.
	Purified water ad	60 mL

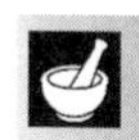

Make isoton. sol.
Sig. One drop in each eye.

Step 1. 60 mL × 0.9% w/v = 0.54 g of sodium chloride or its equivalent needed to prepare 60 mL of an isotonic solution.

Step 2. The quantity of phenacaine hydrochloride required in the prescription is 0.6 g (60 mL × 1% w/v). Then, 0.6 g × 0.20 (*E* value) = 0.12 g of sodium chloride equivalence represented by phenacaine hydrochloride.

The quantity of chlorobutanol required in the prescription is 0.3 g (60 mL × 0.5% w/v). Then, 0.3 g × 0.24 (*E* value) = 0.072 g of sodium chloride equivalence represented by chlorobutanol.

0.12 g + 0.072 g = 0.192 g of sodium chloride equivalence represented by both ingredients.

Step 3. 0.54 g − 0.192 g = 0.348 g of sodium chloride required.

However, because the prescription calls for boric acid and not sodium chloride:

Step 4. 0.348 g ÷ 0.52 (*E* value of boric acid) = 0.669 g of boric acid required.

3. How many grams of sodium chloride should be used in compounding the following prescription?

℞		
	Ingredient X	0.5
	Sodium chloride	q.s.
	Purified water ad	50 mL
	Make isoton. sol.	
	Sig. Eye drops.	

Ingredient X is a new substance for which no sodium chloride equivalent has been previously

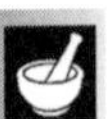

determined. Its molecular weight is 295, and its *i* factor is 2.4.

The sodium chloride equivalent of Ingredient X may be calculated as follows:

$$\frac{58.5}{1.8} \times \frac{2.4}{295} = 0.26$$

Then,

Step 1. 50 mL × 0.9% w/v = 0.45 g of sodium chloride or equivalent required to prepare 50 mL of an isotonic sodium chloride solution.

Step 2. 0.5 g × 0.26 = 0.13 g of sodium chloride equivalence represented by Ingredient X.

Step 3. 0.45 g − 0.13 g = 0.32 g of sodium chloride required.

4. Determine whether each of the following commercial products is hypotonic, isotonic, or hypertonic:

A. An ophthalmic solution containing 40 mg/mL of cromolyn sodium and 0.01% of benzalkonium chloride in purified water
Solving on the basis of 100 mL:

Sodium chloride or equivalent required for isotonicity:

100 mL × 0.9% = 0.9 g

Tonic contribution of cromolyn sodium (*E* value = 0.11):

40 mg/mL × 100 mL = 4,000 mg = 4 g

4 g × 0.11 = 0.44 g

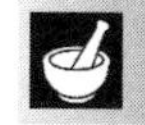

Tonic contribution of benzalkonium chloride (E value = 0.16):

100 mL × 0.01% w/v = 0.01 g
0.01 g × 0.16 = 0.0016 g

Tonic contribution of cromolyn sodium + benzalkonium chloride:

0.44 g + 0.0016 g = 0.4416 g = less than 0.9 g NaCl and therefore hypotonic

B. A parenteral infusion containing 20% w/v of mannitol
Solving on the basis of 100 mL:

Sodium chloride or equivalent required for isotonicity:

100 mL × 0.9% w/v = 0.9 g

Tonic contribution of mannitol (E value = 0.18):

100 mL × 20% w/v = 20 g

20 g × 0.18 = 3.6 g = greater than 0.9 g NaCl and therefore hypertonic

C. A 500-mL large-volume parenteral containing D5W (5%, w/v of anhydrous dextrose in sterile water for injection)
Solving on the basis of 500 mL:

Sodium chloride or equivalent required for isotonicity:

500 mL × 0.9% w/v = 4.5 g

Tonic contribution of anhydrous dextrose (E value = 0.18):

500 mL × 5% w/v = 25 g

25 g × 0.18 = 4.5 g = isotonic

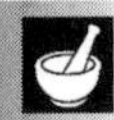

D. A Fleet saline enema containing 19 g of monobasic sodium phosphate, monohydrate, and 7 g of dibasic sodium phosphate, heptahydrate, in 118 mL of aqueous solution Solving on the basis of 118 mL:

Sodium chloride or equivalent required for isotonicity:

118 mL × 0.9% w/v = 1.062 g

Tonic contribution of monobasic sodium phosphate, monohydrate (*E* value = 0.42):

19 g × 0.42 = 7.98 g

Tonic contribution of dibasic sodium phosphate, heptahydrate (*E* value = 0.29):

7 g × 0.29 = 2.03 g

Tonic contribution of monobasic sodium phosphate monohydrate + dibasic sodium phosphate heptahydrate:

7.98 g + 2.03 g = 10.01 g = greater than 1.062 g and therefore hypertonic

5. Calculate the percent concentration of an isotonic solution for a substance having a sodium chloride equivalent of 0.3.

0.9 % ÷ 0.3 = 3%

10

ELECTROLYTE SOLUTIONS

Electrolyte ions in the blood plasma include the cations Na^+, K^+, Ca^{2+}, and Mg^{2+} and the anions Cl^-, HCO_3^-, HPO_4^{2-}, SO_4^{2-}, organic acids, and protein. Electrolyte preparations are used for the treatment of disturbances of the electrolyte and fluid balance in the body.

10.1 Milliequivalents

The milliequivalent is a chemical unit used almost exclusively in the United States to express the concentration of electrolytes in solution.

Definition. The *milliequivalent* is a unit that reflects the chemical activity of an electrolyte based on its valence.

Expression. Milliequivalent units are abbreviated as *mEq*.

Discussion. The milliequivalent weight of a substance can be determined by dividing its molecular weight by its valence. This milliequivalent weight can then be used as a conversion between milligrams and milliequivalents as follows:

$$\text{mg} = \text{mEq} \times \frac{\text{Molecular weight}}{\text{Valence}}$$

$$\text{mEq} = \text{mg} \times \frac{\text{Valence}}{\text{Molecular weight}}$$

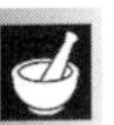

For example, aluminum has a +3 charge, or a valence of 3, and a molecular weight of 27. Carbonate has a –2 charge, or a valence of 2, and a molecular weight of 60. As a result, aluminum carbonate, $Al_2(CO_3)_3$, has a *combined total* valence of 6 and a molecular weight of $(2 \times 27) + (3 \times 60) = 234$. Furthermore, 50 mg of aluminum carbonate would be $50 \text{ mg} \times 6 \text{ mEq}/234 \text{ mg} = 1.28 \text{ mEq}$.

For any given chemical compound, the milliequivalents of the compound are equal to the milliequivalents of the cation (positively charged ion), which are equal to the milliequivalents of the anion (negatively charged ion). This holds true for milliequivalents, but not for the actual weights of the ions. In the example of aluminum carbonate above, 1.28 mEq of aluminum carbonate is equal to 1.28 mEq of aluminum ion, which is equal to 1.28 mEq of carbonate ion. In contrast, 50 mg of aluminum carbonate is not equal to 50 mg of aluminum ion nor 50 mg of carbonate ion.

Key Points. Because the milliequivalent is a measurement of the chemical activity of an electrolyte, the total valence of the cation or anion in the compound must be taken into account. Sodium chloride, for example, has a total valence of one because there is one sodium cation with a +1 charge and one chloride anion with a –1 charge in the compound. However, sodium citrate has a total valence of three because there are three sodium ions with a +1 charge (for a total of +3) and one citrate ion with a –3 charge. Knowing the valence of various compounds is essential in the calculation of milliequivalents.

Pharmacy Applications. The dose for many electrolyte compounds is given based on milliequivalents. Because milliequivalents are a measure of chemical activity and not a quantitative weight measurement, the pharmacist must be able to convert milliequivalents to weight units such as milligrams or grams when preparing a formulation. Furthermore, many drugs are salts and are dosed based on quantitative weight, usually in milligrams. To determine the amount of an ion in chemical activity units received from a dose, the pharmacist must be able to convert the dose to milliequivalents of that ion.

EXAMPLE PROBLEMS

1. What is the concentration, in milligrams per milliliter, of a solution containing 23.5 mEq of sodium chloride per milliliter? (molecular weight of NaCl = 58.5)

$$\frac{23.5 \text{ mEq}}{1 \text{ mL}} \times \frac{58.5 \text{ mg}}{1 \text{ mEq}} = 1{,}374.75 \text{ mg/mL}$$

2. Half-normal saline is 0.45% sodium chloride. Express this concentration in mEq/mL.

$$\frac{0.45 \text{ g}}{100 \text{ mL}} \times \frac{1{,}000 \text{ mg}}{1 \text{ g}} \times \frac{1 \text{ mEq}}{58.5 \text{ mg}} = 0.077 \text{ mEq/mL}$$

3. Trace electrolytes additive (Tracelyte) contains 0.25 mEq of calcium per milliliter. If 20 mL of Tracelyte is included in 1 L of TPN solution, how many milligrams of calcium chloride is this equivalent to? (molecular weight of $CaCl_2$ = 111)

$$0.25 \text{ mEq } Ca^{2+}\text{/mL} = 0.25 \text{ mEq } CaCl_2\text{/mL}$$

$$\frac{0.25 \text{ mEq } CaCl_2}{1 \text{ mL}} \times 20 \text{ mL} \times \frac{111 \text{ mg}}{2 \text{ mEq}} = 277.5 \text{ mg } CaCl_2$$

4. The molecular weight of lithium carbonate, Li_2CO_3, is 73.89. How many milliequivalents of lithium ion are present in a 300-mg tablet of lithium carbonate?

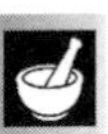

$$300 \text{ mg} \times \frac{2 \text{ mEq}}{73.89 \text{ mg}} = 8.12 \text{ mEq } Li_2CO_3$$

$$= 8.12 \text{ mEq } Li^+$$

5. How many grams of potassium citrate monohydrate powder are needed to prepare 1 L of an oral solution containing 2 mEq of potassium per milliliter? (molecular weight of $K_3C_6H_5O_7 \bullet H_2O$ = 324)

$$2 \text{ mEq } K^+/\text{mL} = 2 \text{ mEq } K_3C_6H_5O_7 \bullet H_2O/\text{mL}$$

$$\frac{2 \text{ mEq}}{1 \text{ mL}} \times 1{,}000 \text{ mL} \times \frac{324 \text{ mg}}{3 \text{ mEq}} \times \frac{1 \text{ g}}{1{,}000 \text{ mg}}$$

$$= 216 \text{ g}$$

6. The following formula will produce 36 lollipop-size "gag tablet" lozenges[1]:

℞		
Sodium chloride	46.56 g	(molecular weight = 58.5)
Potassium chloride	3.00 g	(molecular weight = 74.5)
Calcium lactate	6.12 g	(molecular weight = 218)
Magnesium citrate	2.04 g	(molecular weight = 450)
Sodium bicarbonate	22.44 g	(molecular weight = 84)
Sodium phosphate monobasic	3.84 g	(molecular weight = 120)
Silica gel	3.60 g	
Polyethylene glycol 1,450	40.28 g	

A. How many total milliequivalents of sodium are contained in each lozenge?

$$\text{NaCl: } \frac{46.56\text{ g}}{36\text{ lozenges}} \times \frac{1{,}000\text{ mg}}{1\text{ g}} \times \frac{1\text{ mEq}}{58.5\text{ mg}} = 22.11\text{ mEq Na}^+/\text{lozenge}$$

$$\text{NaHCO}_3\text{: } \frac{22.44\text{ g}}{36\text{ lozenges}} \times \frac{1{,}000\text{ mg}}{1\text{ g}} \times \frac{1\text{ mEq}}{84\text{ mg}} = 7.42\text{ mEq Na}^+/\text{lozenge}$$

$$\text{NaH}_2\text{PO}_4\text{: } \frac{3.84\text{ g}}{36\text{ lozenges}} \times \frac{1{,}000\text{ mg}}{1\text{ g}} \times \frac{1\text{ mEq}}{120\text{ mg}} = 0.89\text{ mEq Na}^+/\text{lozenge}$$

$$\text{Total} = 22.11\text{ mEq/lozenge} + 7.42\text{ mEq/lozenge} + 0.89\text{ mEq/lozenge} = 30.42\text{ mEq Na}^+/\text{lozenge}$$

B. How many milliequivalents each of potassium, calcium, and magnesium are contained in each lozenge?

$$\text{KCl: } \frac{3\text{ g}}{36\text{ lozenges}} \times \frac{1{,}000\text{ mg}}{1\text{ g}} \times \frac{1\text{ mEq}}{74.5\text{ mg}} = 1.12\text{ mEq K}^+/\text{lozenge}$$

$$\text{Ca(C}_3\text{H}_5\text{O}_3)_2\text{: } \frac{6.12\text{ g}}{36\text{ lozenges}} \times \frac{1{,}000\text{ mg}}{1\text{ g}} \times \frac{2\text{ mEq}}{218\text{ mg}} = 1.56\text{ mEq Ca}^{2+}/\text{lozenge}$$

$$\text{Mg}_3\text{(C}_6\text{H}_5\text{O}_7)_2\text{: } \frac{2.04\text{ g}}{36\text{ lozenges}} \times \frac{1{,}000\text{ mg}}{1\text{ g}} \times \frac{6\text{ mEq}}{450\text{ mg}} = 0.76\text{ mEq Mg}^{2+}/\text{lozenge}$$

7. An intravenous solution is prepared using 18 g of ticarcillin disodium (Ticar) diluted to 500 mL with 0.45% sodium chloride and will infuse over 1 day. How many milliequivalents of sodium will the patient receive per day from this infusion?

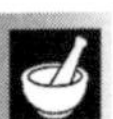

(molecular weight of ticarcillin disodium = 428.43 and valence = 2; assume the drug occupies a negligible volume)

Amount of sodium in drug:

$$\frac{18\text{ g}}{1\text{ day}} \times \frac{1{,}000\text{ mg}}{1\text{ g}} \times \frac{2\text{ mEq}}{428.43\text{ mg}} = 84.03\text{ mEq/day}$$

Amount of sodium in diluent:

$$\frac{500\text{ mL}}{1\text{ day}} \times \frac{0.45\text{ g}}{100\text{ mL}} \times \frac{1{,}000\text{ mg}}{1\text{ g}} \times \frac{1\text{ mEq}}{58.5\text{ mg}} = 38.46\text{ mEq/day}$$

Total amount of sodium:

$$84.03\text{ mEq/day} + 38.46\text{ mEq/day} = 122.49\text{ mEq/day}$$

10.2 Millimoles

The International System (SI), which is used in European countries and in many others throughout the world, expresses electrolyte concentrations in millimoles per liter.

Definition. The *millimole* is a unit that reflects the combining power of a chemical species.

Expression. Millimoles are abbreviated as *mmol.*

Discussion. A mole is the molecular weight of a substance in grams. A millimole is 1/1,000 of the molecular weight in grams, or the molecular weight of a substance in milligrams. This molecular weight can then be used

as a conversion between milligrams and millimoles as follows:

mg = mmol × molecular weight

mmol = mg ÷ molecular weight

Notice that millimolar conversions do not take into account the valence of an ion as do milliequivalent conversions. Therefore, for monovalent species, the numeric value of the milliequivalent and millimole are identical. Using the aluminum carbonate example from Section 10.1, 50 mg of aluminum carbonate would be 50 mg × 1 mmol/234 mg = 0.21 mmol. Similar to milliequivalents, the millimoles of the compound are equal to the millimoles of the cation, which are equal to the millimoles of the anion, but this does not hold true for the actual weights of the ions.

Pharmacy Applications. Milliequivalents are used almost exclusively in the United States to express concentrations of electrolyte ions in a solution; however, millimoles are sometimes used in expressions of clinical laboratory values. Millimoles are also used to express concentrations in some electrolyte solutions when determining the valence of the ions can be quite complicated, such as in the case of the phosphate ion, which can exist in a monovalent ($H_2PO_4^-$), divalent (HPO_4^{2-}), or trivalent (PO_4^{3-}) form.

EXAMPLE PROBLEMS

1. Extra Strength Alka-Seltzer Effervescent Tablets contain 1,985 mg of sodium bicarbonate per tablet. How many millimoles of sodium bicarbonate are contained in each tablet? (molecular weight of $NaHCO_3$ = 84)

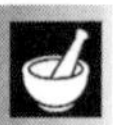

$$\frac{1{,}985\text{ mg}}{1\text{ tablet}} \times \frac{1\text{ mmol}}{84\text{ mg}} = 23.63\text{ mmol/tablet}$$

2. A cardioplegic solution includes 117 mmol/L of potassium chloride and 10 mmol/L of sodium chloride. How many grams of each are required to prepare 5 L of the cardioplegic solution? (molecular weight of KCl = 74.5, molecular weight of NaCl = 58.5)

$$\text{KCl: } \frac{117\text{ mmol}}{1\text{ L}} \times \frac{74.5\text{ mg}}{1\text{ mmol}} \times 5\text{ L} \times \frac{1\text{ g}}{1{,}000\text{ mg}} = 43.58\text{ g}$$

$$\text{NaCl: } \frac{10\text{ mmol}}{1\text{ L}} \times \frac{58.5\text{ mg}}{1\text{ mmol}} \times 5\text{ L} \times \frac{1\text{ g}}{1{,}000\text{ mg}} = 2.93\text{ g}$$

3. The normal range for tobramycin levels is 0.5–2 μg/mL (trough) to 4–8 μg/mL (peak). Convert these ranges to conventional SI units, μmol/L. (molecular weight of tobramycin = 467.52)[2]

$$\frac{0.5\ \mu\text{g}}{1\text{ mL}} \times \frac{1\ \mu\text{mol}}{467.52\ \mu\text{g}} \times \frac{1{,}000\text{ mL}}{1\text{ L}} = 1.07\ \mu\text{mol/L}$$

$$\frac{2\ \mu\text{g}}{1\text{ mL}} \times \frac{1\ \mu\text{mol}}{467.52\ \mu\text{g}} \times \frac{1{,}000\text{ mL}}{1\text{ L}} = 4.28\ \mu\text{mol/L}$$

$$\frac{4\ \mu\text{g}}{1\text{ mL}} \times \frac{1\ \mu\text{mol}}{467.52\ \mu\text{g}} \times \frac{1{,}000\text{ mL}}{1\text{ L}} = 8.56\ \mu\text{mol/L}$$

$$\frac{8\ \mu\text{g}}{1\text{ mL}} \times \frac{1\ \mu\text{mol}}{467.52\ \mu\text{g}} \times \frac{1{,}000\text{ mL}}{1\text{ L}} = 17.11\ \mu\text{mol/L}$$

Tobramycin trough: 1.07–4.28 μmol/L

Tobramycin peak: 8.56–17.11 μmol/L

4. Potassium phosphates injection contains 236 mg potassium phosphate, dibasic (molecular weight =

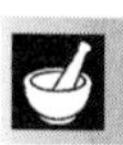

174) and 224 mg potassium phosphate, monobasic (molecular weight = 136) per milliliter. What is the concentration of phosphate (mmol/mL) and potassium (mEq/mL) in this injection?

Phosphate:

Dibasic: $\frac{236\text{ mg}}{1\text{ mL}} \times \frac{1\text{ mmol}}{174\text{ mg}} = 1.36\text{ mmol/mL}$

Monobasic: $\frac{224\text{ mg}}{1\text{ mL}} \times \frac{1\text{ mmol}}{136\text{ mg}} = 1.65\text{ mmol/mL}$

Total: 1.36 mmol/mL + 1.65 mmol/mL

= 3.01 mmol/mL

Potassium:

Dibasic: $\frac{236\text{ mg}}{1\text{ mL}} \times \frac{2\text{ mEq}}{174\text{ mg}} = 2.71\text{ mEq/mL}$

Monobasic: $\frac{224\text{ mg}}{1\text{ mL}} \times \frac{1\text{ mEq}}{136\text{ mg}} = 1.65\text{ mEq/mL}$

Total: 2.71 mEq/mL + 1.65 mEq/mL

= 4.36 mEq/mL

10.3 Milliosmoles and Osmolarity

Osmotic pressure is important to biologic processes that involve the diffusion of solutes or the transfer of fluids through semipermeable membranes, and it is proportional to the total number of particles in solution.

Definition. The *milliosmole* is a unit that reflects the osmotic activity of a substance. *Osmolarity* is an expression of osmotic concentration as milliosmoles per liter.

Expression. Milliosmoles are abbreviated as *mOsmol* or *mOsm*, and units for osmolarity are given as *mOsmol/L* or *mOsm/L*.

Discussion. Because osmotic pressure is proportional to the total number of particles in solution, the units used to measure osmotic concentration must reflect the total number of particles in solution. The milliosmolar weight of a substance can be determined by dividing its molecular weight by the number of species into which it dissociates. This milliosmolar weight can then be used as a conversion between milligrams and milliosmoles as follows:

$$\text{Milligrams} = \text{Milliosmoles} \times \frac{\text{Molecular weight}}{\text{Number of species}}$$

$$\text{Milliosmoles} = \text{Milligrams} \times \frac{\text{Number of species}}{\text{Molecular weight}}$$

For a nonelectrolyte, such as dextrose, the number of species would be one because it does not dissociate. However, for electrolytes the number of ions produced when the compound dissociates must be determined, and in most cases, complete dissociation of the electrolyte can be assumed. Aluminum carbonate will dissociate into two aluminum ions and three carbonate ions, so 50 mg of aluminum carbonate would be 50 mg × 5 mOsmol/234 mg = 1.07 mOsmol.

A distinction also should be made between the terms osmolarity and osmolality. Whereas osmolarity is the milliosmoles of solute per *liter of solution*, osmolality is the number of milliosmoles of solute per *kilogram of solvent*. Osmolarity and osmolality are nearly identical for dilute aqueous solutions, but accurate conversion between the two measurements can only be accomplished by using the specific gravity of the solution. The pharmacist should pay particular attention to a product's label statement regarding osmolarity versus osmolality.

Key Points. Because milliosmoles reflect the osmotic activity of a solution, the milliosmoles of each chemical

in the solution are added to give the total osmolarity. It is critical that the number of ions into which the chemical dissociates be accurately determined in the calculation of osmolarity.

The calculated osmolarity is in most cases slightly higher than the measured osmolarity because of physicochemical interaction among solute particles. For example, the ideal osmolarity of 0.9% sodium chloride injection is:

$$\frac{0.9\ \text{g}}{100\ \text{mL}} \times \frac{1{,}000\ \text{mg}}{1\ \text{g}} \times \frac{1{,}000\ \text{mL}}{1\ \text{L}} \times \frac{2\ \text{mOsmol}}{58.5\ \text{mg}} = 307.69\ \text{mOsmol/L}$$

The actual measured osmolarity of the solution, however, is about 286 mOsmol/L because all sodium chloride ions in solution do not completely dissociate into two ions.

Some pharmaceutical manufacturers label electrolyte solutions with the calculated, or ideal, osmolarities, whereas others list experimental or actual osmolarities. The pharmacist should appreciate this distinction.

Pharmacy Applications. It is important to be able to determine the osmolar concentration of various solutions, especially those prepared for parenteral, ophthalmic, nasal, rectal, or vaginal administration. The labels of intravenous solutions for fluid, nutrient, or electrolyte replenishment and of the osmotic diuretic mannitol are required to state the osmolar concentration. This information indicates to the practitioner whether the solution is hypoosmotic, isoosmotic, or hyperosmotic with regard to biologic fluids and membranes.

Normal serum osmolality is considered to be within the range of 275 to 295 mOsmol/kg, and hyperosmolar infusion solutions may potentially damage the vasculature into which they are infused. The Infusion Nursing Society (INS) recommends that solutions with osmolari-

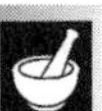

ties greater than 500 mOsmol/L be infused into a central vein to minimize or prevent vascular injury.[3] Hypo-osmolar solutions also may cause problems because of potential lysis of red blood cells; however, most hypo-osmolar solutions are used as diluents and are not usually infused directly.

EXAMPLE PROBLEMS

1. You have a vial of magnesium sulfate solution with a concentration of 4.06 mEq/mL. Express this concentration as mg/mL and mOsmol/L (molecular weight of $MgSO_4$ = 120).

$$\frac{4.06 \text{ mEq}}{1 \text{ mL}} \times \frac{120 \text{ mg}}{2 \text{ mEq}} = 243.6 \text{ mg/mL}$$

$$\frac{243.6 \text{ mg}}{1 \text{ mL}} \times \frac{2 \text{ mOsmol}}{120 \text{ mg}} \times \frac{1{,}000 \text{ mL}}{1 \text{ L}} = 4{,}060 \text{ mOsmol/L}$$

2. What is the osmolarity of a solution containing 5% dextrose and 0.45% sodium chloride? (molecular weight of dextrose = 180, molecular weight of NaCl = 58.5)

$$\frac{5 \text{ g}}{100 \text{ mL}} \times \frac{1{,}000 \text{ mg}}{1 \text{ g}} \times \frac{1 \text{ mOsmol}}{180 \text{ mg}} \times \frac{1{,}000 \text{ mL}}{1 \text{ L}} = 277.78 \text{ mOsmol/L}$$

$$\frac{0.45 \text{ g}}{100 \text{ mL}} \times \frac{1{,}000 \text{ mg}}{1 \text{ g}} \times \frac{2 \text{ mOsmol}}{58.5 \text{ mg}} \times \frac{1{,}000 \text{ mL}}{1 \text{ L}} = 153.85 \text{ mOsmol/L}$$

$$\text{Total} = 277.78 \text{ mOsmol/L} + 153.85 \text{ mOsmol/L} = 431.62 \text{ mOsmol/L}$$

3. Extra Strength Alka-Seltzer Effervescent Tablets contain 1,985 mg of sodium bicarbonate per tablet.

Calculate the osmolarity of a solution produced by placing two Extra Strength Alka-Seltzer Effervescent Tablets in an 8-oz glass of water. (molecular weight of $NaHCO_3$ = 84; assume that 8 oz is the final volume of the solution)

$$\frac{1{,}985\text{ mg}}{1\text{ tablet}} \times 2\text{ tablets} \times \frac{2\text{ mOsmol}}{84\text{ mg}} = 94.52\text{ mOsmol}$$

$$8\text{ oz} \times \frac{29.57\text{ mL}}{1\text{ oz}} = 236.56\text{ mL}$$

$$\frac{94.52\text{ mOsmol}}{236.56\text{ mL}} \times \frac{1{,}000\text{ mL}}{1\text{ L}} = 399.58\text{ mOsmol/L}$$

4. An intravenous solution is prepared using 18 g of ticarcillin disodium (Ticar) diluted to 500 mL with 0.45% sodium chloride and will infuse over 1 day. What would be the osmolarity of this solution? (molecular weight of ticarcillin disodium = 428.43 and dissociates into three ions; assume the drug occupies a negligible volume)

Osmolarity of drug:

$$\frac{18\text{ g}}{500\text{ mL}} \times \frac{1{,}000\text{ mg}}{1\text{ g}} \times \frac{1{,}000\text{ mL}}{1\text{ L}} \times \frac{3\text{ mOsmol}}{428.43\text{ mg}} = 252.08\text{ mOsmol/L}$$

Osmolarity of diluent:

$$\frac{0.45\text{ g}}{100\text{ mL}} \times \frac{1{,}000\text{ mg}}{1\text{ g}} \times \frac{2\text{ mOsmol}}{58.5\text{ mg}} \times \frac{1{,}000\text{ mL}}{1\text{ L}} = 153.85\text{ mOsmol/L}$$

Total osmolarity:

$$252.08\text{ mOsmol/L} + 153.85\text{ mOsmol/L} = 405.93\text{ mOsmol/L}$$

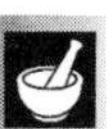

5. A hyperalimentation solution is prepared by mixing 500 mL of 50% dextrose solution and 500 mL of Aminosyn II 8.5% amino acids injection. What would be the osmolarity of this solution? (molecular weight of dextrose = 180, osmolarity of the Aminosyn II 8.5% solution is 742 mOsmol/L[4])

Total volume = 1,000 mL = 1 L

Dextrose:

$$\frac{50 \text{ g}}{100 \text{ mL}} \times 500 \text{ mL} = 250 \text{ g in 1 L of solution}$$

$$\frac{250 \text{ g}}{1 \text{ L}} \times \frac{1{,}000 \text{ mg}}{1 \text{ g}} \times \frac{1 \text{ mOsmol}}{180 \text{ mg}} = 1{,}388.89 \text{ mOsmol/L}$$

Amino acids:

$$\frac{742 \text{ mOsmol}}{1 \text{ L}} \times \frac{1 \text{ L}}{1{,}000 \text{ mL}} \times 500 \text{ mL}$$

$$= 371 \text{ mOsmol in 1 L of solution or } 371 \text{ mOsmol/L}$$

$$\text{Total} = 1{,}388.89 \text{ mOsmol/L} + 371 \text{ mOsmol/L} = 1{,}759.89 \text{ mOsmol/L}$$

References

1. Ford P. Gag tablet. International Journal of Pharmaceutical Compounding 1998;3:46.
2. Prince SJ. Calculations. International Journal of Pharmaceutical Compounding 2001;5:485.
3. Alexander M, ed. Infusion Nursing Standards of Practice. Journal of Intravenous Nursing 2000;23(6S):S37-S38.
4. CliniSphere 2.0 [book on CD-ROM]. St. Louis, MO: Facts and Comparisons, 2002.

C

Patient Parameters and Dosing Calculations

CHAPTER 16 Veterinary Dosing

16.1 Based on Body Weight
16.2 Based on Body Surface Area

CHAPTER 17 Consideration of Drugs Requiring Patient-Specific Dosing

17.1 Aminoglycosides
17.2 Vancomycin
17.3 Digoxin
17.4 Heparin
17.5 Warfarin
17.6 Iron
17.7 Theophylline

11

GENERAL DOSAGE CALCULATIONS

The *dose* of a drug is the amount taken by a patient for the intended therapeutic effect, and the *dosage regimen* is the schedule of dosing for a drug. Many factors contribute to determining the dose and dosage regimen, including potency of the drug and route of administration, as well as patient factors such as weight, disease state, and tolerance. Some drugs may require a *loading* dose to produce an adequate blood level to yield the desired therapeutic effect, then this dose would be followed by smaller *maintenance* doses to maintain an adequate blood level. A *prophylactic* dose of a drug may be given to prevent a disease, but a *therapeutic* dose, which is usually higher than the prophylactic dose, is given to treat an ongoing disease. The dose for most drugs is given in units of weight (i.e., 500 mg), but some drugs, such as biologics, are given based on their activity (i.e., 10 units).

The doses for many drugs, such as antihypertensives, are general and usually not patient-specific. However, the doses for some drugs require patient data such as body surface area (see Section 11.4), pharmacokinetic parameters (see Chapter 12), or clinical laboratory values (see Chapter 17).

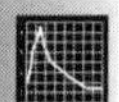

It is the pharmacist's responsibility to ensure that the patient receives the proper dose from his or her medication, and the pharmacist must educate the patient and/or caregiver about the proper measurement of doses. For solid dosage forms, the correct dose is easily administered in premeasured capsules or tablets. However, if the drug is a liquid, the dose is usually a volume that must be accurately measured using a standardized 5-mL teaspoon, calibrated dropper, or syringe. If the pharmacist compounds a specific product for a patient, it is also his or her responsibility to ensure that the correct amount of drug is delivered in each dose.

11.1 Size of Dose, Number of Doses, and Total Amount of Drug

There are different types of information that a pharmacist may need in dealing with dosing problems. The required information can usually be found in one of three categories: size of dose, number of doses, or total amount of drug.

Definitions. *Size of dose* is the quantitative amount needed to deliver the prescribed amount of drug and is usually measured by weight, volume, or dosage units. *Number of doses* is the doses available in a specified quantity, and the *total amount* is the amount of drug or product needed to supply the prescribed dose and dosage regimen.

Discussion. The following equation can be used to calculate any of the aforementioned parameters:

$$\text{Total amount} = \text{Number of doses} \times \text{Size of dose}$$

To properly use this equation, the total amount and the dose must be measured in a common denomination. Dimensional analysis can also be used successfully to determine any of these factors as long as the size of the dose is written as quantitative amount per dose as shown in the following example problems. When calculating the size of the dose, the dose may be rounded to the nearest whole number or to a practical dose depending on the strength of medication available.

EXAMPLE PROBLEMS

1. If the dose of a drug is 50 mg, how many doses will be contained in 0.8 g?

   Using the equation:

   $$\text{Size of dose} = 50\text{ mg} \times \frac{1\text{ g}}{1{,}000\text{ mg}} = 0.05\text{ g}$$

   $$\text{Total amount} = 0.8\text{ g}$$

   $$\text{Number of doses} = \frac{0.8\text{ g}}{0.05\text{ g}} = 16\text{ doses}$$

   Solving by dimensional analysis:

   $$0.8\text{ g} \times \frac{1\text{ dose}}{50\text{ mg}} \times \frac{1{,}000\text{ mg}}{1\text{ g}} = 16\text{ doses}$$

2. If the dose of a medication is 1 and ½ teaspoonsful, how many doses will be contained in 6 fl oz of the medication?

   $$\text{Size of dose} = 1.5\text{ tsp} \times \frac{5\text{ mL}}{1\text{ tsp}} = 7.5\text{ mL}$$

   $$\text{Total amount} = 6\text{ fl oz} \times \frac{29.57\text{ mL}}{1\text{ fl oz}} = 177.42\text{ mL}$$

   $$\text{Number of doses} = \frac{177.42\text{ mL}}{7.5\text{ mL}}$$

   $$= 23.66\text{ doses} \approx 23\text{ full doses}$$

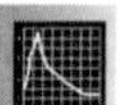

3. What would be the size of each dose if a patient is to take the contents of a 2 fl oz bottle in six divided doses?

Total amount = 2 fl oz

Number of doses = 6

$$\text{Size of dose} = \frac{2 \text{ fl oz}}{6 \text{ doses}} \times \frac{29.57 \text{ mL}}{1 \text{ fl oz}}$$

$$= 9.86 \text{ mL/dose}$$

4. A patient is to receive a total daily dose of 500 mg given in divided doses q.i.d. What is the size of each dose?

$$\frac{500 \text{ mg}}{4 \text{ doses}} = 125 \text{ mg/dose}$$

5. If you need 12 doses of a certain drug, how much drug will you need if the dose is 250 mg?

Number of doses = 12

Size of dose = 250 mg

$$\text{Total amount} = 12 \text{ doses} \times \frac{250 \text{ mg}}{1 \text{ dose}}$$

$$= 3{,}000 \text{ mg} = 3 \text{ g}$$

6. How many milliliters of a solution would you need if the patient is to be taking 1 teaspoonful twice daily for 2 weeks?

$$\frac{1 \text{ tsp}}{1 \text{ dose}} \times \frac{5 \text{ mL}}{1 \text{ tsp}} = 5 \text{ mL/dose}$$

$$\frac{2 \text{ doses}}{1 \text{ day}} \times \frac{7 \text{ days}}{1 \text{ week}} \times 2 \text{ weeks} = 28 \text{ doses}$$

$$\frac{5 \text{ mL}}{1 \text{ dose}} \times 28 \text{ doses} = 140 \text{ mL}$$

7. How much of a solution would you need to dispense if the directions to the patient are “ii gtts

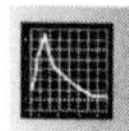

q6h x 4 d"? The drop factor for the dropper is 25 gtts/mL.

$$\frac{2 \text{ gtts}}{1 \text{ dose}} \times \frac{1 \text{ mL}}{25 \text{ gtts}} = 0.08 \text{ mL/dose}$$

$$\frac{4 \text{ doses}}{1 \text{ day}} \times 4 \text{ days} = 16 \text{ doses}$$

$$\frac{0.08 \text{ mL}}{1 \text{ dose}} \times 16 \text{ doses} = 1.28 \text{ mL}$$

8. If 500 mg of drug are used to prepare 90 mL of a syrup, how much drug is contained in each teaspoonful dose?

$$\frac{500 \text{ mg}}{90 \text{ mL}} \times \frac{1 \text{ tsp}}{1 \text{ dose}} \times \frac{5 \text{ mL}}{1 \text{ tsp}} = 27.78 \text{ mg/dose}$$

9. If 60 g of a drug are used to prepare 200 capsules, what is the daily dose of the drug if the dosage regimen is one capsule three times daily?

$$\frac{60 \text{ g}}{200 \text{ capsules}} \times \frac{1 \text{ capsule}}{1 \text{ dose}} \times \frac{3 \text{ doses}}{1 \text{ day}} = 0.9 \text{ g/day}$$

10. How many milligrams of codeine sulfate and of ammonium chloride will be contained in each dose of the following prescription?

℞		
℞	Codeine sulfate	0.6 g
	Ammonium chloride	6 g
	Cherry syrup q.s. ad.	120 mL

Sig: ʒ i qid for cough

Remember that the dram sign in the sig denotes "teaspoonful," which is 5 mL.

$$\text{Codeine sulfate: } \frac{0.6 \text{ g}}{120 \text{ mL}} \times \frac{5 \text{ mL}}{1 \text{ dose}} \times \frac{1{,}000 \text{ mg}}{1 \text{ g}} = 25 \text{ mg/dose}$$

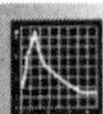

$$\text{Ammonium chloride: } \frac{6\text{ g}}{120\text{ mL}} \times \frac{5\text{ mL}}{1\text{ dose}} \times \frac{1{,}000\text{ mg}}{1\text{ g}} = 250\text{ mg/dose}$$

11. A certain compounded prescription calls for 10 mg of drug in each teaspoonful dose. How much drug is required to prepare 4 oz of this liquid?

$$\frac{10\text{ mg}}{1\text{ tsp}} \times \frac{1\text{ tsp}}{5\text{ mL}} \times \frac{29.57\text{ mL}}{1\text{ oz}} \times 4\text{ oz} = 236.56\text{ mg}$$

12. A physician asks the pharmacist to compound codeine sulfate tablet triturates containing 10 mg of codeine. The patient needs a 5-day supply and may take 1–2 q4–6h prn. How much codeine is needed to fill this prescription?

When figuring a dose of a drug as given above, always consider that the patient might be taking the maximum amount of the drug. Therefore, this patient could be taking two tablets per dose and six doses per day.

$$\frac{10\text{ mg}}{1\text{ tablet}} \times \frac{2\text{ tablets}}{1\text{ dose}} \times \frac{6\text{ doses}}{1\text{ day}} \times 5\text{ days} = 600\text{ mg}$$

11.2 Dosing Based on Age

Pediatric and geriatric patients require special dosing considerations because of many factors. Most dosage adjustments for geriatric patients are attributable to age-related decline of physiologic functions. On the other hand, pediatric patients usually weigh less than an adult patient, and certain body systems may not be fully developed. Many times the only dosing information avail-

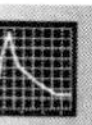

able is for adult dosages; therefore, the pediatric dose must be calculated based on the adult dose given. This dose can be calculated based on the child's age, weight, or body surface area.

Discussion. Calculating the dosage based on age is somewhat inaccurate because this method does not take into account that children's weights and sizes vary greatly within an age group. However, if the only information available is the child's age, then these equations may prove useful.

Young's rule:

$$\frac{\text{Age (in years)}}{\text{Age} + 12} \times \text{Adult dose} = \text{Dose for child}$$

Cowling's rule:

$$\frac{\text{Age at next birthday (in years)} \times \text{Adult dose}}{24} = \text{Dose for child}$$

Fried's rule for infants:

$$\frac{\text{Age (in months)} \times \text{Adult dose}}{150} = \text{Dose for infant}$$

Currently, when age *is* considered in determining dosage of a *potent* therapeutic agent, it is used generally in conjunction with another factor, such as weight as shown in drug-specific calculations in Chapter 17. In contrast, over-the-counter medications purchased for self-medication include labeling instructions that provide guidelines for safe and effective dosing. For pediatric use, doses generally are based on age groupings, for example, 2 to 6 years old, 6 to 12 years old, and older than 12 years of age. For children 2 years of age or younger, the label recommendation generally states "consult your physician."

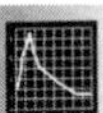

EXAMPLE PROBLEMS

1. The usual adult dose of paroxetine (Paxil) is 20 mg/day for the treatment of obsessive compulsive disorder. What would be the dose for an 11-year-old child? (Use Young's rule)

$$\frac{11}{11 + 12} \times 20 \text{ mg/day} = 9.57 \text{ mg/day}$$

2. The usual adult dose of rofecoxib (Vioxx) is 25 mg/day. What would be the dose for a 6-year-old child? (Use Cowling's rule)

$$\frac{7 \times 25 \text{ mg/day}}{24} = 7.29 \text{ mg/day}$$

3. The usual initial dose for irbesartan (Avapro) is 150 mg daily. What would be the dose for a 7-year-old child? (Use Young's rule)

$$\frac{7}{7 + 12} \times 150 \text{ mg/day} = 55.26 \text{ mg/day}$$

4. The usual adult dose of sparfloxacin (Zagam) is two 200-mg tablets on the first day of therapy followed by one 200-mg tablet daily for the next 9 days. What would be the dosage regimen for a 9-year-old child? (Use Cowling's rule)

$$\frac{10 \times 400 \text{ mg/day}}{24} = 166.67 \text{ mg/day on the first day}$$

$$\frac{10 \times 200 \text{ mg/day}}{24} = 83.33 \text{ mg/day for the next 9 days}$$

5. The usual adult dose of fexofenadine (Allegra) is 60 mg twice daily, for a total dose of 120 mg/day. What would be the dose for a 5-month-old infant?

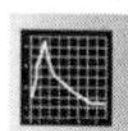

$$\frac{5 \times 60 \text{ mg}}{150}$$

$= 2$ mg twice daily for a total dose of 4 mg/day

6. The usual adult dose of gatifloxacin (Tequin) for bacterial infections is 400 mg/day. What would be the dose for an 8-month-old infant?

$$\frac{8 \times 400 \text{ mg/day}}{150} = 21.33 \text{ mg/day}$$

11.3 Dosing Based on Weight

The *usual doses* for drugs are considered generally suitable for 70-kg (154-lb) individuals. The ratio between the amount of drug administered and the size of the body influences the drug concentration at its site of action. Therefore, drug dosage may require adjustment from the usual adult dose for abnormally lean or obese patients.

Discussion. If the weight for a pediatric patient is available, calculating the dose based on weight would be more appropriate because this method considers the size of the child rather than just the age. Clark's rule, shown below, is a general rule for calculating a pediatric dose based on an adult dose.

Clark's rule:

$$\frac{\text{Weight (in lb)} \times \text{Adult dose}}{150} = \text{Dose for child}$$

Some drugs must be dosed based on each patient's specific body weight. In these instances, the dose of the drug is given in an amount per weight measurement. The specific dose for the patient is then calculated by multiplying the amount/weight dose by the patient's body weight.

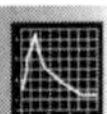

EXAMPLE PROBLEMS

1. The usual adult dose for celecoxib (Celebrex) is 100 mg twice daily, for a total dose of 200 mg/day. How much should a child weighing 52 lb receive per dose?

$$\frac{52 \times 100 \text{ mg}}{150} = 34.67 \text{ mg twice daily}$$

for a total dose of 69.34 mg/day

2. The adult dose for hydrochlorothiazide is 50 mg daily. What would be the dose for a 40-kg child?

$$40 \text{ kg} \times \frac{2.2 \text{ lb}}{1 \text{ kg}} = 88 \text{ lb}$$

$$\frac{88 \times 50 \text{ mg}}{150} = 29.33 \text{ mg/day}$$

3. The usual dose for a drug is 10 mg/kg. How many milligrams should be administered to a patient weighing 125 lb? How many 500-mg tablets should be given?

$$\frac{10 \text{ mg}}{1 \text{ kg}} \times \frac{1 \text{ kg}}{2.2 \text{ lb}} \times 125 \text{ lb} = 568.18 \text{ mg}$$

$$568.18 \text{ mg} \times \frac{1 \text{ tablet}}{500 \text{ mg}} = 1.14 \text{ tablets} \approx 1 \text{ tablet}$$

4. The usual dose of loracarbef (Lorabid) for pharyngitis or tonsillitis in children up to 6 years of age is 15 mg/kg/day in divided doses administered every 12 hours. What would be the dosage regimen for a 4-year-old child weighing 36 lb?

$$\frac{15 \text{ mg}}{1 \text{ kg/day}} \times \frac{1 \text{ kg}}{2.2 \text{ lb}} \times 36 \text{ lb} = 245.45 \text{ mg/day}$$

$$\frac{245.45 \text{ mg}}{1 \text{ day}} \times \frac{1 \text{ day}}{2 \text{ doses}} = 122.73 \text{ mg every 12 hours}$$

5. The maintenance dose of ranitidine for active duodenal and gastric ulcers in children is 2 to 4

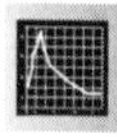

mg/kg once daily. What would be the dosage range for a child weighing 57 lb?

$$\frac{2 \text{ mg}}{1 \text{ kg}} \times \frac{1 \text{ kg}}{2.2 \text{ lb}} \times 57 \text{ lb} = 51.82 \text{ mg}$$

$$\frac{4 \text{ mg}}{1 \text{ kg}} \times \frac{1 \text{ kg}}{2.2 \text{ lb}} \times 57 \text{ lb} = 103.64 \text{ mg}$$

The dosage range would be 51.82–103.64 mg daily.

6. The intramuscular dose of lorazepam is 0.05 mg/kg up to a maximum of 4 mg. How many milliliters of a 4 mg/mL injection should be administered to a 144-lb patient?

$$\frac{0.05 \text{ mg}}{1 \text{ kg}} \times \frac{1 \text{ kg}}{2.2 \text{ lb}} \times 144 \text{ lb} = 3.27 \text{ mg}$$

$$3.27 \text{ mg} \times \frac{1 \text{ mL}}{4 \text{ mg}} = 0.82 \text{ mL}$$

11.4 Dosing Based on Body Surface Area

The *body surface area* (BSA) method of calculating drug doses provides results that are widely used in two types of patient groups: (1) cancer patients receiving chemotherapy, and (2) pediatric patients of all childhood ages, with the exception of premature and full-term newborns, whose immature renal and liver functions require additional assessment in dosing.

Discussion. The most accurate method of calculating a dose is based on the patient's BSA because it takes into account the height and weight of the patient. The patient's BSA can be calculated using the Du Bois and Du Bois formula as follows:[1]

$$S = W^{0.425} \times H^{0.725} \times 71.84$$

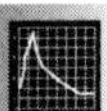

where S = body surface area in cm^2,
W = weight in kg, and H = height in cm

This formula, however, is somewhat difficult to use, and in most instances the BSA must be converted to square meters. The nomograms found in Appendix C are based on the Du Bois and Du Bois formula and are much easier and more efficient to use than the equation. Notice that there are separate nomograms for children and adults, and the height and weight columns are given in both the common and metric systems of measurement. An option to nomograms is the use of the equation shown below:

$$\text{BSA } (m^2) = \sqrt{\frac{\text{Height (cm)} \times \text{Weight (kg)}}{3{,}600}}$$

This equation simplifies the Du Bois and Du Bois formula and is commonly used in practice for the calculation of BSA.

Dosage adjustments can be made based on a patient's BSA using an average adult BSA of 1.73 m^2; therefore, the dose for an adult or child can be estimated using the following equation:

$$\frac{\text{BSA } (m^2)}{1.73 \text{ } m^2} \times \text{Usual adult dose} = \text{Approximate dose}$$

The dose of some drugs is based on each patient's specific BSA, and the dose of the drug is given in an amount per BSA measurement, usually square meters. The specific dose for the patient is then calculated by multiplying the dose per square meter by the patient's BSA.

EXAMPLE PROBLEMS

1. The usual adult dose of a drug is 150 mg. How much should be given to a child who weighs 55 lb and is 3′5″ tall?

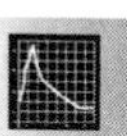

$3'5'' = 41''$

BSA from nomogram in Appendix C = $0.82\ m^2$

$$\frac{0.82\ m^2}{1.73\ m^2} \times 150\ mg = 71.1\ mg$$

2. The adult dose of captopril is 12.5 to 50 mg t.i.d. What would be the dosage range for an adult who is 6′2″ and weighs 270 lb?

BSA from nomogram in Appendix C = $2.48\ m^2$

$$\frac{2.48\ m^2}{1.73\ m^2} \times 12.5\ mg = 17.92\ mg$$

$$\frac{2.48\ m^2}{1.73\ m^2} \times 50\ mg = 71.68\ mg$$

The dosage range should be 17.92–71.68 mg three times daily.

3. Nancy Smith is a 7-year-old female patient who is 3′4″ tall and weighs 37 lb. The pediatrician writes an order for omeprazole (Prilosec) for Nancy and gives instructions for the pharmacist to calculate an appropriate dose. Because the adult dose for omeprazole is 20 mg daily, what should be the dose for Nancy? (Use the BSA equation.)

$$\text{Height} = 40\ in \times \frac{2.54\ cm}{1\ in} = 101.6\ cm$$

$$\text{Weight} = 37\ lb \times \frac{1\ kg}{2.2\ lb} = 16.82\ kg$$

$$\text{BSA} = \sqrt{\frac{101.6\ cm \times 16.82\ kg}{3{,}600}}$$

$$= \sqrt{0.47} = 0.69\ m^2$$

$$\frac{0.69\ m^2}{1.73\ m^2} \times 20\ mg = 7.96\ mg/day$$

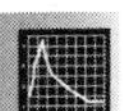

4. If the usual dose of a chemotherapeutic drug is 2.2 mg/m^2, how much should be given to an adult who is 5′7″ and weighs 130 lb? The drug is available as an injectable solution with a concentration of 750 μg/mL. What volume should this patient receive for each dose?

BSA from nomogram = $1.69\ m^2$

$2.2\ mg/m^2 \times 1.69\ m^2 = 3.72\ mg$

$$3.72\ mg \times \frac{1{,}000\ \mu g}{1\ mg} \times \frac{1\ mL}{750\ \mu g} = 4.96\ mL$$

5. An intravenous leucovorin dose of 20 mg/m^2 followed by an intravenous fluorouracil dose of 425 mg/m^2 can be used in the treatment of advanced colorectal carcinoma. What is the dose of these two drugs for an adult who is 5′2″ and weighs 145 lb? (Use the BSA equation.)

$$\text{Height} = 62\ in \times \frac{2.54\ cm}{1\ in} = 157.48\ cm$$

$$\text{Weight} = 145\ lb \times \frac{1\ kg}{2.2\ lb} = 65.91\ kg$$

$$\text{BSA} = \sqrt{\frac{157.48\ cm \times 65.91\ kg}{3{,}600}}$$

$$= \sqrt{2.88} = 1.7\ m^2$$

Leucovorin: $20\ mg/m^2 \times 1.7\ m^2 = 33.96\ mg$

Fluorouracil: $425\ mg/m^2 \times 1.7\ m^2 = 721.64\ mg$

6. Research on a new pediatric drug has shown an effective dose of 40 mg daily given to a child who is 0.9 m tall and weighs 28 kg. What is this daily dosage in mg/m^2?

BSA from nomogram = $0.77\ m^2$

$$\frac{40\ mg/day}{0.77\ m^2} = 51.95\ mg/m^2/day$$

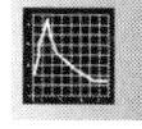

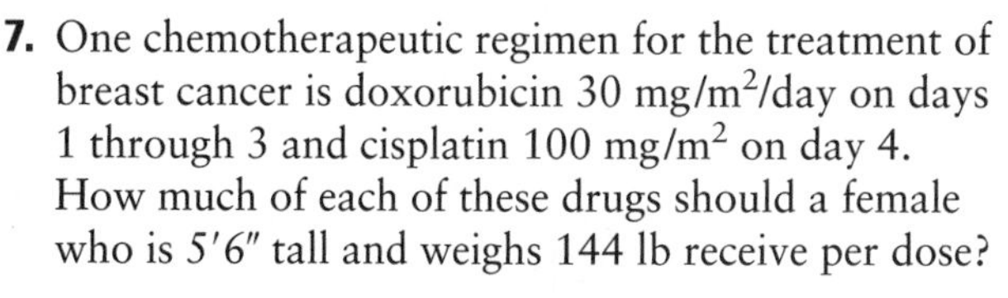

7. One chemotherapeutic regimen for the treatment of breast cancer is doxorubicin 30 mg/m^2/day on days 1 through 3 and cisplatin 100 mg/m^2 on day 4. How much of each of these drugs should a female who is 5′6″ tall and weighs 144 lb receive per dose?

BSA from nomogram = 1.74 m^2

Doxorubicin: 30 mg/m^2/day × 1.74 m^2 = 52.2 mg/day

Cisplatin: 100 mg/m^2 × 1.74 m^2 = 174 mg

8. A dose of cyclophosphamide greater than 1,500 mg/m^2 is 90% likely to cause nausea and vomiting. What would this dose be for a patient who is 4′10″ tall and weighs 134 lb? (Use the BSA equation.)

$$\text{Height} = 58 \text{ in} \times \frac{2.54 \text{ cm}}{1 \text{ in}} = 147.32 \text{ cm}$$

$$\text{Weight} = 134 \text{ lb} \times \frac{1 \text{ kg}}{2.2 \text{ lb}} = 60.91 \text{ kg}$$

$$\text{BSA} = \sqrt{\frac{147.32 \text{ cm} \times 60.91 \text{ kg}}{3{,}600}} = \sqrt{2.49} = 1.58 \text{ m}^2$$

1,500 mg/m^2 × 1.58 m^2 = 2,368.16 mg

Reference

1. Du Bois D, Du Bois EF. A formula to estimate the approximate surface area if height be known. Archives of Internal Medicine 1916;17:863.

12 BASIC PHARMACOKINETICS

Pharmacokinetics is the study and characterization of the time course of the absorption, distribution, metabolism, and excretion (ADME) of drugs. Absorption deals with uptake of the drug from its site of administration into the systemic circulation, or more simply, it addresses how the drug gets into the body. Distribution refers to the transfer of the drug from the blood to extravascular fluids and tissues, or where the drug goes in the body. Metabolism deals with enzymatic or biochemical transformation of the drug to metabolic products, and excretion is the final elimination of the drug from the body through the urine, feces, sweat, and so on.

There are many aspects of pharmacokinetics, and a few of them will be dealt with in this chapter. The reader should consult a pharmacokinetics textbook for a more detailed explanation of this area of study.

12.1 Blood Concentration Versus Time Curves

To construct a blood concentration versus time curve for a drug, a certain dosage form would be administered to

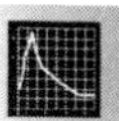

a group of patients, and blood samples would be drawn at determined time periods. These blood samples would then be analyzed for the amount of drug, and a graph of blood concentration versus time would be constructed, such as the one shown in Figure 12-1.

Definitions. Blood concentration versus time curves can be used to determine or present the following parameters:

- Minimum effective concentration (MEC)—the minimum blood concentration of a drug that can be expected to produce the desired effects in a patient

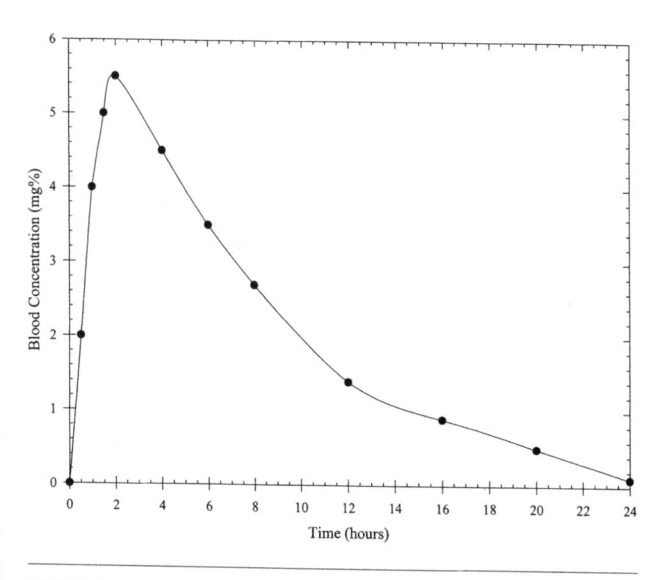

FIGURE 12-1. Example of a blood level curve for a hypothetical drug as a function of the time after oral administration.

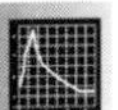

- Minimum toxic concentration (MTC)—the lowest blood concentration of a drug that produces dose-related toxic effects
- Therapeutic window—the difference between the MTC and the MEC
- Onset of action—the time for the blood level to reach the MEC
- Duration of action—the amount of time the blood level remains at or above the MEC
- Peak/maximum concentration (C_{max})—the highest concentration the drug reaches in the blood
- Time to peak/maximum concentration (T_{max})—the time for the blood level to reach the C_{max}
- Area under the curve (AUC)—the total area formed under the blood concentration versus time curve from the initial dose to final elimination of the drug from the body

Expressions. MEC, MTC, therapeutic window, and C_{max} are expressed in units of serum concentration (i.e., mg/dL). T_{max} and onset and duration of action are expressed in units of time. AUC is usually expressed in units of concentration per unit time (i.e., mg/dL/hr).

Discussion. The MEC and MTC are established in clinical studies, then these values are used to find the therapeutic window and onset and duration of action. Using the graph in Figure 12-1 and given an MEC of 3 mg% and an MTC of 5.8 mg%, the parameters listed above can be determined. The therapeutic window is calculated as the MTC minus the MEC, or 5.8 mg% − 3 mg% = 2.8 mg%. The onset of action occurs where

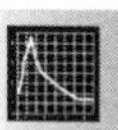

the graphed blood concentration first crosses the MEC, which would be 45 minutes for this particular graph, and the duration of action is read from the horizontal axis where the blood concentration crosses the MEC when increasing and decreasing, which would be 6 hours, 15 minutes. Furthermore, the C_{max} for the drug shown in Figure 12-1 is 5.5 mg% and the T_{max} is 2 hours. Calculation of the AUC is quite complicated and is often determined using a pharmacokinetics software program; therefore, it is outside the scope of this discussion.

Pharmacy Applications. Blood concentration versus time curves are essential for the determination of the proper dose and dosage regimen for a drug. The therapeutic window reflects the safety of a drug because a narrow therapeutic window indicates that the blood level required to produce a desired effect is near the blood level that will produce a toxic effect; therefore, a small variation in the amount absorbed into the bloodstream may cause adverse effects to occur. In addition, the C_{max} and T_{max} can be used to establish a protocol for blood level measurements in a clinical setting for dose adjustments in drugs such as the aminoglycoside antibiotics.

EXAMPLE PROBLEM

Patients were administered a 60-mg tablet of an experimental drug, and blood samples were drawn at certain intervals. These blood samples were analyzed for drug concentration and are reported in graphical form below. The MEC for the drug is 0.55 mmol/L, and the MTC is 1.09 mmol/L.

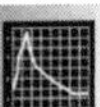

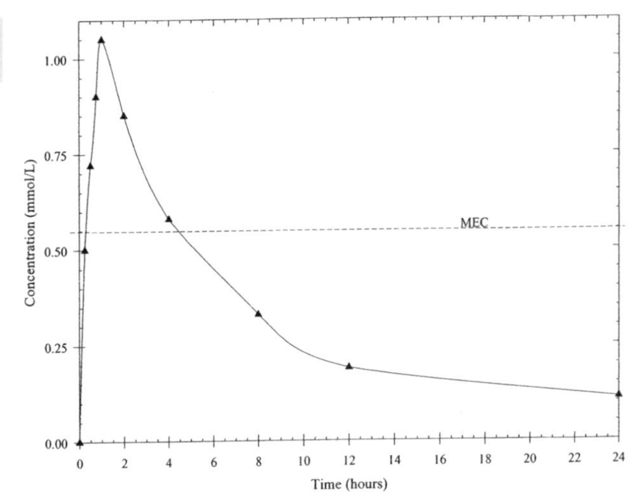

What is the onset of action?
Approximately 20 minutes

What is the duration of action?
The concentration falls below the MEC at approximately 4 hours, 30 minutes, so the duration of action would be 4 hours, 30 minutes − 20 minutes = 4 hours, 10 minutes

What is the C_{max}?
1.05 mmol/L

What is the T_{max}?
1 hour

What is the therapeutic window?
1.09 mmol/L − 0.55 mmol/L = 0.54 mmol/L

12.2 Bioavailability and Bioequivalence

Definitions. The *bioavailability* of a drug is based on the amount of drug that actually reaches the blood-

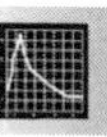

stream from an administered dosage form. Two or more drugs are considered *bioequivalent* if their rate and extent of absorption do not show a significant difference when administered at the same dose under similar experimental conditions.

Discussion. The bioavailability of a drug varies with the dosage form; for example, digoxin is 100% bioavailable in the intravenous (IV) form, 90% to 100% bioavailable in the capsule form, 70% to 85% bioavailable in the elixir form, and 60% to 80% bioavailable in the tablet form.[1] Therefore, the bioavailability is determined using the AUC of the blood concentration versus time curve for a particular dosage form of a drug. The bioavailability is usually expressed as the bioavailability factor (F) and is calculated using the following equation:

$$F = \frac{AUC_{\text{Dosage form}}}{AUC_{IV}}$$

The AUC for the IV form is used because none of the drug is lost due to absorption when it is injected directly into the bloodstream. The bioavailability factor can be used to adjust the dose when changing from one dosage form to another with the following equation:

$$F_A Dose_A = F_B Dose_B$$

where F_A and F_B are the bioavailability factors for dosage forms A and B, respectively, and $Dose_A$ and $Dose_B$ are the doses for the drug in dosage forms A and B, respectively.

The dosage regimen must be taken into account in this calculation because it may be different for the dosage forms. For example, estradiol tablets are taken once daily, but estradiol patches are applied every 3 to 4 days. Therefore, the total daily dose should be used and then divided into doses for the dosage form required.

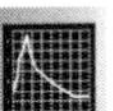

Bioequivalence is affected by the absorption of the drug and is established by comparing the blood concentration versus time curves for the drugs under consideration. The C_{max}, T_{max}, and AUC are used in evaluating whether different drug formulations are bioequivalent.

Pharmacy Applications. On dismissal from the hospital, a patient may be switched from parenteral medications to oral or topical medications for self-care at home. Therefore, the bioavailabilities of the dosage forms under consideration can be used in switching this patient to a more convenient dosage form.

Bioequivalence is used in determining effective brand-name medication to generic medication substitutions as well as comparisons of different salt or ester forms of drugs.

EXAMPLE PROBLEMS

1. The AUC for an oral dose of a drug is 4.5 μg/mL/hr and for an IV dose is 11.2 μg/mL/hr. What is the bioavailability of an oral dose of this drug?

$$F = \frac{AUC_{oral}}{AUC_{IV}} = \frac{4.5\ \mu g/mL/hr}{11.2\ \mu g/mL/hr} = 0.4 \text{ or } 40\%$$

2. A patient has been receiving ranitidine (Zantac) 50 mg q8h IV. The person now needs to switch to the oral liquid form of the drug to leave the hospital. The oral liquid form is 50% bioavailable, is supplied in a strength of 75 mg/tsp, and should be taken b.i.d. How many milliliters of ranitidine syrup should be given for each dose?

$$\text{IV daily dose} = \frac{50\ mg}{1\ dose} \times \frac{3\ doses}{1\ day} = 150\ mg/day$$

F for the IV route is 1 or 100%

$100\% \times 150 \text{ mg/day} = 50\% \times \text{Dose}_{\text{oral}}$

$\text{Dose}_{\text{oral}} = 300 \text{ mg/day}$

$$\frac{300 \text{ mg}}{1 \text{ day}} \times \frac{1 \text{ day}}{2 \text{ doses}} = 150 \text{ mg/dose}$$

$$\frac{150 \text{ mg}}{1 \text{ dose}} \times \frac{5 \text{ mL}}{75 \text{ mg}} = 10 \text{ mL/dose}$$

3. A drug is 40% bioavailable by the oral route and 58% bioavailable by the transdermal route. If a patient is taking a 2.5 mg capsule b.i.d. and decides to switch to the 2% ointment, how many grams of the ointment should be administered daily to provide the same dose?

$$\text{Oral daily dose} = \frac{2.5 \text{ mg}}{1 \text{ dose}} \times \frac{2 \text{ doses}}{1 \text{ day}} = 5 \text{ mg/day}$$

$40\% \times 5 \text{ mg/day} = 58\% \times \text{Dose}_{\text{oint}}$

$\text{Dose}_{\text{oint}} = 3.45 \text{ mg/day}$

$$\frac{3.45 \text{ mg drug}}{1 \text{ day}} \times \frac{100 \text{ g ointment}}{2 \text{ g drug}} \times \frac{1 \text{ g}}{1{,}000 \text{ mg}} = 0.17 \text{ g ointment daily}$$

4. An orally administered drug used to treat asthma is 55% bioavailable. The patient is currently taking 5 mg daily and wishes to switch to the inhalational form of the drug, which is 87% bioavailable. How many sprays of the drug in inhalational form should the patient use every 12 hours if each metered spray delivers 500 μg of drug?

$55\% \times 5 \text{ mg/day} = 87\% \times \text{Dose}_{\text{inh}}$

$\text{Dose}_{\text{inh}} = 3.16 \text{ mg/day}$

$$\frac{3.16 \text{ mg}}{1 \text{ day}} \times \frac{1 \text{ day}}{2 \text{ doses}} \times \frac{1{,}000 \text{ μg}}{1 \text{ mg}} \times \frac{1 \text{ spray}}{500 \text{ μg}} = 3.16 \text{ sprays/dose} \approx 3 \text{ sprays/dose}$$

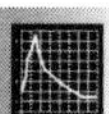

12.3 Protein Binding of Drugs

When a drug is absorbed into the bloodstream, some of it may be bound to proteins in the blood and some will remain unbound. The amount of drug that is bound to proteins will affect the distribution and elimination of the drug.

Definition. Protein binding reflects the amount of drug that is covalently bound to albumin and other proteins in the blood.

Discussion. The amount of unbound drug is expressed as the fraction symbolized by the Greek letter α and is calculated using the following equation:

$$\alpha = \frac{C_U}{C_U + C_B} = \frac{C_U}{C_T}$$

where C_U is the plasma concentration of unbound drug, C_B is the plasma concentration of bound drug, and C_T is the total plasma concentration of the drug.

The equation above can also be used to determine the amount of unbound drug if the total amount of drug in plasma and α are known. The free or unbound portion of drug is available for transport to its site of action in the tissues to produce a clinical effect. The unbound portion of drug is also more readily available for elimination than the bound portion. Therefore, the amount of drug that is unbound will greatly affect its activity and duration of action, and a change in this free drug amount will cause a change in its effects. Drug reference sources often report the percent of drug that is protein bound rather than stating α for a drug. The α value can be determined from the percent protein bound by subtracting the percent as a decimal fraction from one, or

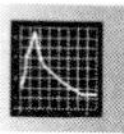

$\alpha = 1 - (\%\text{ protein bound}/100)$. For example, phenytoin is reported to be 87% to 93% protein bound,[1] which corresponds to $\alpha = 0.07 - 0.13$.

Pharmacy Applications. Protein binding is the primary cause of interactions for some drugs because of the impact one drug may have on the protein-binding of another. A classic example of this problem is warfarin, which is approximately 99% protein bound.[1] Any drug that may displace warfarin from protein binding sites and decrease the protein-bound portion by only 1% will double the amount of free warfarin in the bloodstream, which can lead to a dangerous overdose. Therefore, it is imperative that the pharmacist understands the implications of protein binding.

EXAMPLE PROBLEMS

1. If, at equilibrium, two-thirds of the amount of a drug substance in the blood is bound to protein, what would be the α value of the drug?

If two-thirds of the drug is bound, then one-third is unbound. Or, one drug molecule out of every three molecules is unbound.

Therefore, $\alpha = \frac{1}{3} = 0.333$

2. The serum concentration of a drug is analyzed and found to be 0.4 μg/mL. You look in the drug product literature and find that the α value for the drug is 0.22. What is the plasma concentration of free drug?

$$0.22 = \frac{C_U}{0.4\ \mu g/mL}$$

$$C_U = 0.22 \times 0.4\ \mu g/mL = 0.088\ \mu g/mL$$

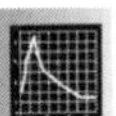

3. The serum concentration of phenytoin is found to be 28 μg/mL and is approximately 90% protein bound. What is the plasma concentration of free drug?

$$\alpha = 1 - \frac{90}{100} = 0.1$$

$$0.1 = \frac{C_U}{28\ \mu g/mL}$$

$$C_U = 0.1 \times 28\ \mu g/mL = 2.8\ \mu g/mL$$

12.4 Volume of Distribution

Definition. *Apparent volume of distribution* (Vd) is a hypothetical volume of body fluid that would be required to dissolve the total amount of drug at the same concentration as that found in the blood.

Expression. Volume of distribution is usually expressed in liters.

Discussion. From the definition above, it can be stated that the blood or plasma concentration of a drug (C_P) would be equal to the amount of drug injected intravenously (D) divided by its volume of distribution (Vd). This concept is better stated in equation form as follows:

$$C_P = \frac{D}{Vd}$$

This equation can be rearranged to answer a number of questions, as shown in the following problems. Only drugs administered intravenously will be considered here because addressing the amount of drug lost in the absorption process is outside the scope of this overview.

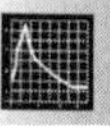

Pharmacy Applications. The volume of distribution will vary for each patient; therefore, this parameter can be used to determine doses or dosage adjustments to produce the desired blood levels in individual patients.

EXAMPLE PROBLEMS

1. A 6-mg dose is administered IV and produces a blood concentration of 0.4 μg/mL. What is its volume of distribution?

$$\frac{0.4\ \mu g}{1\ mL} = \frac{6\ mg}{Vd}$$

$$Vd = 6\ mg \times \frac{1\ mL}{0.4\ \mu g} \times \frac{1{,}000\ \mu g}{1\ mg} \times \frac{1\ L}{1{,}000\ mL} = 15\ L$$

2. The patient in Example Problem 1 starts showing signs of overdose after a second dose of the drug. A blood sample is analyzed and found to contain 0.65 μg/mL of the drug. Assuming that all of the drug from the first dose had been excreted before the patient received the second dose, and the patient's clinical status (e.g., weight and hydration) remained stable, how much drug did the patient receive in the second dose?

$$\frac{0.65\ \mu g}{1\ mL} = \frac{D}{15\ L}$$

$$D = \frac{0.65\ \mu g}{1\ mL} \times 15\ L \times \frac{1{,}000\ mL}{1L} \times \frac{1\ mg}{1{,}000\ \mu g} = 9.75\ mg$$

3. The serum concentration of phenytoin is measured at 15 μg/mL after a 100-mg IV dose. What is its volume of distribution?

$$\frac{15\ \mu g}{1\ mL} = \frac{100\ mg}{Vd}$$

$$Vd = 100\ mg \times \frac{1\ mL}{15\ \mu g} \times \frac{1{,}000\ \mu g}{1\ mg} \times \frac{1\ L}{1{,}000\ mL} = 6.67\ L$$

4. The volume of distribution of a drug is 11.4 L. What serum concentration would an IV dose of 30 mg produce?

$$C_P = \frac{30\ mg}{11.4\ L} \times \frac{1{,}000\ \mu g}{1\ mg} \times \frac{1\ L}{1{,}000\ mL} = 2.63\ \mu g/mL$$

12.5 Elimination Rate Constant and Half-Life

As a drug is excreted from the body via the feces, urine, or other body fluids, its concentration in the blood will decrease accordingly.

Definitions. The *elimination rate constant* (K_{el}) is the fractional rate of drug removal per unit time, and the *elimination half-life* ($t_{1/2}$) is the time for the plasma concentration (C_P) to decrease to one-half of its original value.

Expression. The elimination rate constant is expressed as a decimal fraction with units of inverse time (i.e., 0.01 min^{-1}). The elimination half-life is expressed in units of time.

Discussion. The K_{el} can be calculated from the slope of the line formed on a graph of plasma concentration versus time plotted as a semilogarithmic graph. This

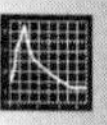

value can then be used to calculate the half-life by using the following equation:

$$t_{1/2} = \frac{0.693}{K_{el}}$$

The half-life can also be determined directly from a graph of plasma concentration versus time by choosing a concentration and establishing the amount of time for the plasma concentration to decrease by half. For example, if the initial plasma concentration is 5 mg/L, the amount of time it takes for the plasma concentration to reach 2.5 mg/L would be the elimination half-life. If in this case $t_{1/2}$ = 4 hours and C_P = 5 mg/L at 8:00 AM, then at 12:00 PM C_P = 2.5 mg/L, 4:00 PM C_P = 1.25 mg/L, 8:00 PM C_P = 0.625 mg/L, and so on.

Pharmacy Applications. After three to five half-lives, a drug has been eliminated to the extent that it has little or no effect on the body and has decreased to below detectable levels. Therefore, the elimination half-life is useful in determining when a drug that may interact with a drug previously given can be administered safely to a patient. It can also be useful in predicting the length of time a drug can be detected for drug abuse screening tests.

EXAMPLE PROBLEMS

1. The elimination rate constant for a drug is 0.58 hour^{-1}. What is the half-life?

$$t_{1/2} = \frac{0.693}{0.58\ \text{hr}^{-1}} = 1.19\ \text{hr}$$

2. The half-life of warfarin is 1 to 2.5 days. What is the elimination rate constant?

$$K_{el} = \frac{0.693}{1\ \text{day}} = 0.69\ \text{day}^{-1}$$

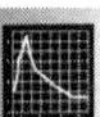

$$K_{el} = \frac{0.693}{2.5 \text{ days}} = 0.28 \text{ day}^{-1}$$

$0.28 - 0.69 \text{ day}^{-1}$

3. Using the information in Example Problem 2 above, calculate the amount of time that warfarin can be detected in the bloodstream after a dose.

$5 \times 1 \text{ day} = 5 \text{ days}$

$5 \times 2.5 \text{ days} = 12.5 \text{ days}$

$5 - 12.5 \text{ days}$

4. The elimination rate constant for a certain drug is 2.7 days^{-1}. What is the half-life?

$$t_{1/2} = \frac{0.693}{2.7 \text{ days}^{-1}} = 0.26 \text{ day} \times \frac{24 \text{ hours}}{1 \text{ day}}$$
$$= 6.16 \text{ hours}$$

Reference

1. CliniSphere 2.0 [book on CD ROM]. St. Louis, MO: Facts and Comparisons, 2002.

13

DETERMINATION AND EVALUATION OF PATIENT PARAMETERS

In the practice of pharmacy, it is often necessary to determine and evaluate various patient parameters. These parameters can then be used, for example, to calculate appropriate doses or to determine a patient's nutritional status.

13.1 Ideal Body Weight

The *ideal body weight* (IBW) is useful in determining the loading and maintenance doses of many drugs.

Definition. The IBW is the goal weight of a patient based on his or her height.

Expression. IBW is expressed in kilograms or pounds.

Discussion. The IBW is often used in calculating doses when the patient's body weight cannot or should not be used. The following equations based on the patient's

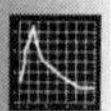

height and gender can be used to calculate IBW for an adult:

For males:

IBW (kg) = 50 kg + 2.3 kg for each inch of patient's height over 5 feet

IBW (lb) = 110 lb + 5 lb for each inch over 5 feet

For females:

IBW (kg) = 45.5 kg + 2.3 kg for each inch of patient's height over 5 feet

IBW (lb) = 100 lb + 5 lb for each inch over 5 feet

To calculate IBW of children 1 to 18 years old, the following equation can be used:[1]

$$\text{IBW (kg)} = \frac{(\text{height in cm})^2 \times 1.65}{1{,}000}$$

A patient is considered to be of normal weight if his or her actual body weight falls within 30% of the calculated IBW.[2] Adjusted body weight may be used in determining doses for obese patients and is calculated based on the patient's IBW and actual body weight (ABW) as follows:[1]

$$\text{Adjusted weight} = [(\text{ABW} - \text{IBW}) \times 0.2] + \text{IBW}$$

EXAMPLE PROBLEMS

1. What is the IBW (in pounds and kilograms) for a 34-year-old male who is 6′4″ tall?

76″ (6′4″) −60″ (5′) = 16″

IBW = 50 kg + 2.3 kg × 16 in = 86.8 kg

IBW = 110 lb + 5 lb × 16 in = 190 lb

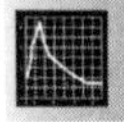

2. What is the IBW (in pounds and kilograms) for a 55-year-old female who is 5′2″ tall?

$$\text{IBW} = 45.5\ \text{kg} + 2.3\ \text{kg} \times 2\ \text{in} = 50.1\ \text{kg}$$

$$\text{IBW} = 100\ \text{lb} + 5\ \text{lb} \times 2\ \text{in} = 110\ \text{lb}$$

3. What is the IBW for a 6-year-old child who is 3′4″ tall?

$$3'4'' = 40''$$

$$40\ \text{in} \times \frac{2.54\ \text{cm}}{1\ \text{in}} = 101.6\ \text{cm}$$

$$\text{IBW} = \frac{(101.6\ \text{cm})^2 \times 1.65}{1{,}000} = 17.03\ \text{kg}$$

4. Calculate the adjusted body weight, in kilograms, for a 38-year-old male weighing 385 lb and measuring 5′8″ tall.

$$\text{IBW} = 50\ \text{kg} + 2.3\ \text{kg} \times 8\ \text{in} = 68.4\ \text{kg}$$

$$\text{ABW} = 385\ \text{lb} \times \frac{1\ \text{kg}}{2.2\ \text{lb}} = 175\ \text{kg}$$

$$\text{Adjusted weight} = [(175\ \text{kg} - 68.4\ \text{kg}) \times 0.2] + 68.4\ \text{kg} = 89.72\ \text{kg}$$

13.2 Body Mass Index

Body mass index (BMI) is accepted as the clinical standard for judging excessive weight and obesity.

Definition. BMI is defined as body weight in kilograms divided by the square of height measured in meters.

Expression. BMI is usually expressed without units; however, the understood units are kg/m^2.

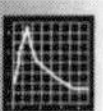

Discussion. BMI can be determined from a table such as the one shown in Figure 13-1. It also can be calculated using the following formula:

$$BMI = \frac{\text{Weight (kg)}}{[\text{Height (m)}]^2}$$

According to the National Institutes of Health (NIH),[3] individuals with a BMI:

- Less than 18.5 may be considered underweight;
- 18.5 to 24.9 may be considered weight-normal;
- 25 to 29.9 are considered overweight;

WEIGHT

HEIGHT	100	110	120	130	140	150	160	170	180	190	200	210	220	230	240	250
5'0"	20	21	23	25	27	29	31	33	35	37	39	41	43	45	47	49
5'1"	19	21	23	25	26	28	30	32	34	36	38	40	42	43	45	47
5'2"	18	20	22	24	26	27	29	31	33	35	37	38	40	42	44	46
5'3"	18	19	21	23	25	27	28	30	32	34	35	37	39	41	43	44
5'4"	17	19	21	22	24	26	27	29	31	33	34	36	38	39	41	43
5'5"	17	18	20	22	23	25	27	28	30	32	33	35	37	38	40	42
5'6"	16	18	19	21	23	24	26	27	29	31	32	34	36	37	39	40
5'7"	16	17	19	20	22	23	25	27	28	30	31	33	34	36	38	39
5'8"	15	17	18	20	21	23	24	26	27	29	30	32	33	35	36	38
5'9"	15	16	18	19	21	22	24	25	27	28	30	31	32	34	35	37
5'10"	14	16	17	19	20	22	23	24	26	27	29	30	32	33	34	36
5'11"	14	15	17	18	20	21	22	24	25	26	27	28	30	32	33	35
6'0"	14	15	16	18	19	20	22	23	24	26	27	28	30	31	33	34
6'1"	13	15	16	17	18	20	21	22	24	25	26	28	29	30	32	33
6'2"	13	14	15	17	18	19	21	22	23	24	26	27	28	30	31	32
6'3"	12	14	15	16	17	19	20	21	22	24	25	26	27	29	30	31
6'4"	12	13	15	16	17	18	19	21	22	23	24	26	27	28	29	30

BMI interpretation

- Underweight: under 18.5
- Normal: 18.5–24
- Overweight: 25–29.9
- Obese: 30 and over

FIGURE 13-1. Table used to determine body mass index. (Reprinted with permission from Ansel HC, Stoklosa MJ. Pharmaceutical Calculations. 11th Ed. Baltimore, MD: Lippincott Williams & Wilkins, 2001:227.)

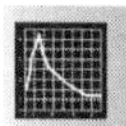

- 30 and above are considered obese; and
- Greater than 40 are considered extremely obese.

Pharmacy Applications. Distribution into fat tissue may be considered in the dosing of some drugs (e.g., aminoglycoside antibiotics); therefore, BMI may assist in determining whether a patient is obese and requires weight-based dose adjustments of such drugs. Furthermore, obesity may contribute to many chronic diseases, including hypertension, heart disease, and type 2 diabetes mellitus. Therefore, it is important for the pharmacist to be able to calculate BMI to determine obesity so that he or she may be able to intervene and improve a patient's quality of life.

EXAMPLE PROBLEMS

1. Calculate the BMI of a person 4′11″ in height and weighing 98 lb.

$$98 \text{ lb} \times \frac{1 \text{ kg}}{2.2 \text{ lb}} = 44.55 \text{ kg}$$

$$4'11'' = 59 \text{ in}$$

$$59 \text{ in} \times \frac{2.54 \text{ cm}}{1 \text{ in}} \times \frac{1 \text{ m}}{100 \text{ cm}} = 1.5 \text{ m}$$

$$\text{BMI} = \frac{44.55 \text{ kg}}{(1.5 \text{ m})^2} = 19.83$$

2. Calculate the BMI of a person 6′0″ in height and weighing 182 lb.

$$182 \text{ lb} \times \frac{1 \text{ kg}}{2.2 \text{ lb}} = 82.73 \text{ kg}$$

$$6'0'' = 72 \text{ in}$$

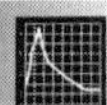

$$72 \text{ in} \times \frac{2.54 \text{ cm}}{1 \text{ in}} \times \frac{1 \text{ m}}{100 \text{ cm}} = 1.83 \text{ m}$$

$$\text{BMI} = \frac{82.73 \text{ kg}}{(1.83 \text{ m})^2} = 24.74$$

13.3 Lean Body Mass

Definition. *Lean body mass* (LBM) is the energy-utilizing component of body weight excluding skeletal mass and body fat.

Expression. LBM is expressed in kilograms or pounds.

Discussion. LBM represents both structural and functional proteins. An accurate determination of LBM would require the measurement of visceral proteins, which include albumin, prealbumin, transferrin, and retinol-binding protein, as well as measurement of skeletal muscle mass using midarm-muscle circumference.[1] The measurement of visceral proteins, however, is impractical and can be greatly affected by disease states such as renal insufficiency and dehydration. Therefore, a useful estimation of LBM can be made using the following formula[4]:

For males:

$$\text{LBM (kg)} = [1.10 \times \text{Weight(kg)}] - 128\left\{\frac{[\text{Weight(kg)}]^2}{[100 \times \text{Height(m)}]^2}\right\}$$

For females:

$$\text{LBM (kg)} = [1.07 \times \text{Weight(kg)}] - 148\left\{\frac{[\text{Weight(kg)}]^2}{[100 \times \text{Height(m)}]^2}\right\}$$

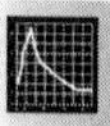

Because LBM includes only the energy-utilizing component of the body, such as muscle mass, it is useful in evaluating a patient's nutritional needs.

EXAMPLE PROBLEMS

1. Calculate the LBM of a 45-year-old male who is 5′8″ tall and weighs 195 lb.

$$\text{Height} = 5'8'' = 68 \text{ in} \times \frac{2.54 \text{ cm}}{1 \text{ in}} \times \frac{1 \text{ m}}{100 \text{ cm}} = 1.73 \text{ m}$$

$$\text{Weight} = 195 \text{ lb} \times \frac{1 \text{ kg}}{2.2 \text{ lb}} = 88.64 \text{ kg}$$

$$\text{LBM} = [1.10 \times 88.64 \text{ kg}] - 128\left\{\frac{[88.64 \text{ kg}]^2}{[100 \times 1.73 \text{ m}]^2}\right\} = 63.79 \text{ kg}$$

2. Calculate the LBM of a 79-year-old female who is 5′1″ tall and weighs 88 lb.

$$\text{Height} = 5'1'' = 61 \text{ in} \times \frac{2.54 \text{ cm}}{1 \text{ in}} \times \frac{1 \text{ m}}{100 \text{ cm}} = 1.55 \text{ m}$$

$$\text{Weight} = 88 \text{ lb} \times \frac{1 \text{ kg}}{2.2 \text{ lb}} = 40 \text{ kg}$$

$$\text{LBM} = [1.07 \times 40 \text{ kg}] - 148\left\{\frac{[40 \text{ kg}]^2}{[100 \times 1.55 \text{ m}]^2}\right\} = 32.94 \text{ kg}$$

13.4 Creatinine Clearance

Creatinine is a biochemical product of muscle metabolism and is eliminated from the body through the kidneys. The amount of creatinine in the blood is used to

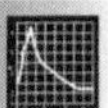

determine *creatinine clearance* (CrCl), which is a measurement of a patient's kidney function and an estimate of actual glomerular filtration rate.

Definition. The creatinine clearance rate represents the volume of blood plasma that is cleared of creatinine by kidney filtration per minute.

Expression. Creatinine clearance is usually expressed in milliliters per minute.

Discussion. Because creatinine is eliminated from the body essentially through renal filtration, reduced kidney performance causes an increase in serum creatinine because of reduced creatinine clearance rate. The normal adult range of serum creatinine is 0.7 to 1.5 mg/dL, and serum creatinine values above 1.5 mg/dL indicate renal insufficiency. The Cockcroft-Gault equation[5] is most commonly used in calculating creatinine clearance because it takes into account the patient's serum creatinine, body weight, gender, and age, as shown below:

For males:

$$\text{CrCl(mL/min)} = \frac{(140 - \text{age in years}) \times \text{Body weight in kg}}{72 \times \text{Serum creatinine in mg/dL}}$$

For females:

$$\text{CrCl} = 0.85 \times \text{CrCl for males}$$

This equation, however, may be inaccurate in patients who are obese or who have rapidly declining renal function; therefore, a more detailed analysis of renal function may be in order. In some cases it may be necessary to adjust the patient's creatinine clearance for body surface area to account for this possible variable in determining

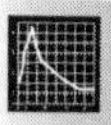

drug dosage. This requires obtaining the patient's body surface area (see Section 11.4) and the formula below:

$$\frac{\text{BSA}(\text{m}^2)}{1.73\ \text{m}^2} \times \text{CrCl} = \text{Adjusted CrCl}$$

Pharmacy Applications. Creatinine clearance is important because many drugs are eliminated by the kidneys. If a patient's kidney function declines, the elimination rate for drugs excreted in the urine will also decrease and cause a corresponding increase in the plasma concentration. A significant increase in plasma concentration can cause the drug to reach toxic levels; therefore, the dose may need to be adjusted to account for the reduced elimination of the drug.

EXAMPLE PROBLEMS

1. What is the creatinine clearance for a 68-year-old female weighing 160 lb and having a serum creatinine of 1.8 mg/dL?

$$160\ \text{lb} \times \frac{1\text{kg}}{2.2\ \text{lb}} = 72.73\ \text{kg}$$

$$\text{CrCl} = 0.85 \times \frac{(140 - 68\ \text{yr}) \times 72.73\ \text{kg}}{72 \times 1.8\ \text{mg/dL}}$$

$$= 34.34\ \text{mL/min} \approx 34\ \text{mL/min}$$

2. If the patient in Example Problem 1 above is 5′8″ tall, what would be the adjusted creatinine clearance?

BSA (from nomogram in Appendix C) = $1.86\ \text{m}^2$

$$\frac{1.86\ \text{m}^2}{1.73\ \text{m}^2} \times 34.34\ \text{mL/min}$$

$$= 36.92\ \text{mL/min} \approx 37\ \text{mL/min}$$

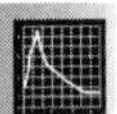

3. What is the creatinine clearance for a 75-year-old male weighing 185 lb and having a serum creatinine concentration of 0.97 mg/dL?

$$185 \text{ lb} \times \frac{1 \text{ kg}}{2.2 \text{ lb}} = 84.09 \text{ kg}$$

$$\text{CrCl} = \frac{(140 - 75 \text{ yr}) \times 84.09 \text{ kg}}{72 \times 0.97 \text{ mg/dL}}$$
$$= 78.26 \text{ mL/min} \approx 78 \text{ mL/min}$$

4. What is the creatinine clearance for a 35-year-old female who is 5′7″ tall, weighs 234 lb, and has a serum creatinine concentration of 7.2 mg/dL?

$$234 \text{ lb} \times \frac{1 \text{ kg}}{2.2 \text{ lb}} = 106.36 \text{ kg}$$

$$\text{CrCl} = 0.85 \times \frac{(140 - 35 \text{ yr}) \times 106.36 \text{ kg}}{72 \times 7.2 \text{ mg/dL}}$$
$$= 18.31 \text{ mL/min} \approx 18 \text{ mL/min}$$

Note: The patient's body weight is greater than 130% of her IBW; therefore, the Cockcroft-Gault equation may be inaccurate for this patient.

13.5 Resting Metabolic Energy and Total Daily Calories

The caloric requirements for patients will vary depending on their physical state and medical condition. Therefore, it is imperative that the pharmacist be able to determine the caloric requirements to assess proper nutritional support for a patient.

Definition. The *resting metabolic energy* (RME) estimates the amount of energy needed to maintain basic bodily functions (e.g., heartbeat, breathing, metabolism).

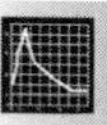

RME is also known as *basal energy expenditure* (BEE). *Total daily calories* (TDC) is the amount of nutrition needed to maintain the patient's current weight based on disease state and level of activity.

Expression. RME and TDC are usually expressed in units of kilocalories per day (kcal/day).

Discussion. Calculation of patient-specific RME can be accomplished using the Harris-Benedict equations below[6]:

For males:

$$RME = 66 + (13.7 \times W) + (5 \times H) - (6.8 \times A)$$

For females:

$$RME = 655 + (9.6 \times W) + (1.8 \times H) - (4.7 \times A)$$

where W is the patient's weight in kilograms, H is height in centimeters, and A is age in years.

Because the caloric need estimated by the RME only accounts for maintenance of bodily functions, the patient's actual nutritional need is usually greater than the RME. Therefore, in most cases the RME is multiplied by an activity factor or stress factor to determine the patient's TDC as follows:[7]

No stress or mild stress (i.e., normal activity or mild trauma): RME × 1.2 to 1.3
Moderate stress (i.e., moderate sepsis or moderate to severe trauma): RME × 1.3 to 1.5
Severe stress (i.e., severe sepsis or burns): RME × 1.6 to 2.0

The TDC may be further adjusted based on the patient's clinical and nutritional status.

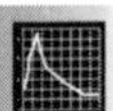

Pharmacy Applications. The pharmacist must consider the caloric needs of a patient to supply the appropriate enteral or parenteral nutrition support (see Chapter 15). Proper nutritional support is essential to aiding a patient in improving his or her disease status.

EXAMPLE PROBLEMS

1. Using the Harris-Benedict equation and assuming no stress factor, calculate the RME for a 58-year-old female who is 5′3″ tall and weighs 140 lb.

$$A = 58 \text{ yr}$$

$$H = 5'3'' = 63 \text{ in} \times \frac{2.54 \text{ cm}}{1 \text{ in}} = 160.02 \text{ cm}$$

$$W = 140 \text{ lb} \times \frac{1 \text{ kg}}{2.2 \text{ lb}} = 63.64 \text{ kg}$$

$$\text{RME} = 655 + (9.6 \times 63.64) + (1.8 \times 160.02) - (4.7 \times 58) = 1{,}281.35 \text{ kcal/day}$$

2. Calculate the total daily calories for a 76-year-old male who is 6′2″, weighs 201 lb, and has suffered mild trauma because of a fracture of his femur. Use the Harris-Benedict equation and a stress factor of 1.2.

$$A = 76 \text{ yr}$$

$$H = 6'2'' = 74 \text{ in} \times \frac{2.54 \text{ cm}}{1 \text{ in}} = 187.96 \text{ cm}$$

$$W = 201 \text{ lb} \times \frac{1 \text{ kg}}{2.2 \text{ lb}} = 91.36 \text{ kg}$$

$$\text{RME} = 66 + (13.7 \times 91.36) + (5 \times 187.96) - (6.8 \times 76) = 1{,}740.68 \text{ kcal/day}$$

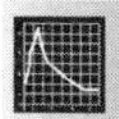

TDC = 1,740.68 kcal/day × 1.2

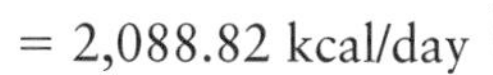

= 2,088.82 kcal/day

3. Using the Harris-Benedict equation, what would the caloric requirements be for a severely stressed (use average factor), 28-year-old female who is 5′5″ tall and weighs 132 lb?

A = 28 yr

$$H = 5'5'' = 65 \text{ in} \times \frac{2.54 \text{ cm}}{1 \text{ in}} = 165.1 \text{ cm}$$

$$W = 132 \text{ lb} \times \frac{1 \text{ kg}}{2.2 \text{ lb}} = 60 \text{ kg}$$

$$RME = 655 + (9.6 \times 60) + (1.8 \times 165.1) - (4.7 \times 28) = 1{,}396.58 \text{ kcal/day}$$

Stress factor = 1.6 to 2.0, average = 1.8

TDC = 1,396.58 kcal/day × 1.8

= 2,513.84 kcal/day

References

1. Dipiro JT, Talbert RL, Yee GC, et al, eds. Pharmacotherapy: A Pathophysiologic Approach. 5th Ed. New York, NY: McGraw-Hill, 2002:2447–2450.
2. Dipiro JT, Talbert RL, Yee GC, et al, eds. Pharmacotherapy: A Pathophysiologic Approach. 5th Ed. New York, NY: McGraw-Hill, 2002:41.
3. Clinical Guidelines on the Identification, Evaluation, and Treatment of Overweight and Obesity in Adults. Bethesda, MD: National Heart, Lung, and Blood Institute, National Institutes of Health, 1996. Available at: http://www.nhlbi.nih.gov/guidelines/obesity/ob_tbl2.htm. Accessed September 5, 2002.
4. Online Clinical Calculator. Milwaukee, WI: Division of General Internal Medicine, Medical College of Wisconsin,

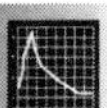

1999. Available at: http://www.intmed.mcw.edu/clincalc/body.htm. Accessed April 11, 2002.

5. Cockcroft DW, Gault MH. Prediction of creatinine clearance from serum creatinine. Nephron 1976;16:31.
6. Harris JA, Benedict FG. A Biometric Study of Basal Metabolism in Man. Publication 279. Washington, DC: Carnegie Institution of Washington, 1919:190, 227.
7. Dipiro JT, Talbert RL, Yee GC, et al, eds. Pharmacotherapy: A Pathophysiologic Approach. 5th Ed. New York, NY: McGraw-Hill, 2002:2456.

14 DOSING CONSIDERATIONS FOR PARENTERAL MEDICATIONS

Parenteral medications are given by injection and include intravenous, intramuscular, subcutaneous, intrathecal, and intra-arterial routes of administration. These medications, therefore, must meet strict standards on sterility and osmolarity. Furthermore, because these medications are injected directly into the tissues or bloodstream, any miscalculation may cause serious adverse consequences.

14.1 Reconstitution of Injectable Powders

Many medications are supplied as powders that are intended to be reconstituted into solutions or suspensions for injection. Such solid dosage forms are preferred for drugs that are unstable in liquid form to extend their shelf life.

Definition. *Reconstitution* is addition of diluent to a concentrated liquid or powder to bring it to a specified concentration.

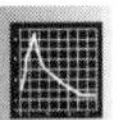

Expression. The labeling on most powders for reconstitution states the amount of diluent to add in milliliters to reach a certain concentration, usually expressed in milligrams per milliliter.

Discussion. When reconstituting a powder, the pharmacist must add the correct volume of water. An error in the amount of water would change the intended concentration, which could produce an overdose or underdose of the medication. On the other hand, the amount of water added to reconstitute powders for injection may not always be critical when the total amount of drug in the vial is administered as one dose. In some cases, a simple fraction of the total amount of drug is given, such as 1 g out of a 2-g vial; therefore, half of the volume would be administered.

The bulk volume of the dry contents of a vial is usually small and may or may not contribute to the final volume of the constituted solution. If the volume of powder *does* contribute significantly to the final volume of the solution, the powder volume must be taken into account. This is especially the case in vials containing several doses of a medication. Manufacturer labels on parenteral powders for reconstitution usually display the total amount of drug in the vial, and the amount of water to add and resulting volume and concentration may be given on the label or package insert. To obtain the volume occupied by the powder, the volume of diluent to be added is subtracted from the final volume after reconstitution. An important concept to keep in mind is that the volume of powder does not change; therefore, producing a concentration other than that given on the label is not a simple dilution problem. For example, a certain drug powder for reconstitution produces a total volume of 10 mL and a concentration of 10 mg/mL when 7 mL of diluent are added. The volume occupied

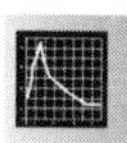

by the powder, then, is 10 mL − 7 mL = 3 mL. If a concentration of 5 mg/mL is desired, simply doubling the volume of diluent to be added would not produce the correct concentration. The total volume of the solution would double (20 mL), but the amount of diluent to be added would be 20 mL − 3 mL = 17 mL.

Key Points. The pharmacist must carefully observe the label directions for reconstituted powders for injection to prepare the correct concentration of drug. The volume of powder must be considered if it contributes significantly to the total volume of the solution.

EXAMPLE PROBLEMS

1. How many milliliters of sterile water for injection should be added to a 2-g vial of aztreonam (Azactam) to get a final concentration of 100 mg/mL?

Lacking further information, it can be assumed that the drug occupies a negligible volume.

$$2\text{ g} \times \frac{1{,}000\text{ mg}}{1\text{g}} \times \frac{1\text{ mL}}{100\text{ mg}} = 20\text{ mL}$$

2. A physician orders penicillin G potassium 400,000 units IM q6h. The dose needs to be administered in a 1-mL volume to cause as little pain to the patient as possible. The following information is available on the package insert for a 5,000,000-unit vial:

"Preparation of solution: Add 18 mL of diluent for a final concentration of 250,000 U/mL."

How much diluent must be added to the vial to make the strength required?

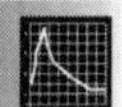

$$\text{Total volume} = 5{,}000{,}000 \text{ units} \times \frac{1 \text{ mL}}{250{,}000 \text{ units}}$$

$$= 20 \text{ mL}$$

Volume occupied by powder

$$= 20 \text{ mL} - 18 \text{ mL} = 2 \text{ mL}$$

$$5{,}000{,}000 \text{ units} \times \frac{1 \text{ mL}}{400{,}000 \text{ units}} = 12.5 \text{ mL total}$$

volume to produce desired concentration

$$12.5 \text{ mL} - 2 \text{ mL} = 10.5 \text{ mL water to add}$$

3. A hospital pharmacist receives the following order:

Nafcillin sodium 800 mg in 100 mL NS

The pharmacist uses a 1-g vial of nafcillin with label directions as follows:

"When reconstituted with 3.4 mL of diluent, each vial contains 4 mL of solution."

However, he reconstitutes the vial with 5 mL of sterile water instead of 3.4 mL as directed on the label. How much of the solution should be added to 100 mL of normal saline for the required dose?

Volume occupied by powder

$$= 4 \text{ mL} - 3.4 \text{ mL} = 0.6 \text{ mL}$$

Total volume mistakenly diluted

$$= 5 \text{ mL} + 0.6 \text{ mL} = 5.6 \text{ mL}$$

$$800 \text{ mg} \times \frac{1 \text{ g}}{1{,}000 \text{ mg}} \times \frac{5.6 \text{ mL}}{1 \text{ g}} = 4.48 \text{ mL}$$

4. A vial containing 6 g of an antibiotic drug for injection has the following directions on the label:

"Add 8.6 mL of sterile water for injection for a final concentration of 1 g/2 mL."

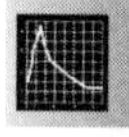

You realize after checking the technician's work that he added 6.8 mL of water to the vial rather than the 8.6 mL as stated on the label. What would be the concentration (in mg/mL) of the solution prepared by the technician?

$$\text{Total volume} = 6\text{ g} \times \frac{2\text{ mL}}{1\text{ g}} = 12\text{ mL}$$

Volume of powder = 12 mL − 8.6 mL = 3.4 mL

Total volume mistakenly diluted

= 6.8 mL + 3.4 mL = 10.2 mL

$$\text{Concentration} = \frac{6\text{ g}}{10.2\text{ mL}} \times \frac{1{,}000\text{ mg}}{1\text{ g}}$$

$$= 588.24\text{ mg/mL}$$

5. The directions for cefamandole (Mandol) for IM injection are as follows:

> "Reconstitute each gram of cefamandole with 3 mL of one of the following diluents: sterile water for injection, bacteriostatic water for injection, 0.9% sodium chloride injection or bacteriostatic sodium chloride injection."

What would be the final concentration of a 2-g vial of cefamandole if reconstituted according to the directions?

$$\text{Volume of diluent to add} = 2\text{ g} \times \frac{3\text{ mL}}{1\text{ g}} = 6\text{ mL}$$

$$\text{Concentration of solution} = \frac{2\text{ g}}{6\text{ mL}} \times \frac{1{,}000\text{ mg}}{1\text{ g}}$$

$$= 333.33\text{ mg/mL}$$

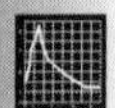

14.2 Intravenous Admixtures

Medications for IV administration are usually available in small-volume vials that are mixed in a large-volume solution by the pharmacist before administration to the patient.

Definition. The solution produced by diluting a drug in a large-volume solution for IV administration is termed an *IV admixture.*

Expression. The drug added to a parenteral solution is often available in a solution. Therefore, the additive amount is calculated in terms of volume, usually milliliters.

Discussion. The amount of drug in a parenteral solution is clearly stated on the label, but the pharmacist must be careful to notice whether the amount is given in terms of concentration (e.g., 10 mg/mL) or amount of drug in the vial (e.g., 80 mg in a 2-mL vial). The concentration is used to calculate the correct volume to be mixed with a parenteral diluent to produce the prescribed dose. In most instances, the dose of the drug is given in units of weight or activity (i.e., mg or mEq), and the dose is then divided by the concentration of the additive solution to calculate the correct volume to be used in the IV admixture. The reader may need to refer to Section 4.1 for a discussion on percentage strength and Section 10.1 for a discussion on milliequivalents.

The total volume of an admixture after preparation should also be considered in some cases. Many times the volume of additive solution is small compared with the volume of diluent solution, and the additive volume is considered to be insignificant. Large-volume parenteral solution containers also have overfill, which makes determination of the exact concentration of a drug in an IV admixture practically impossible. However, for drug solutions that should be prepared as a specific concentration, the exact volumes of the additive and diluent solutions must be accurately measured using a large-volume syringe. Many hospital pharmacies have protocols for which medications need to be mixed as exact volumes, and these procedures, therefore, allow for accurate administration of the drugs from container to container.

Key Points. When preparing an IV admixture, the pharmacist must read the strength of drug carefully to determine the amount of solution needed to prepare the admixture. Once a drug has been given intravenously, it is taken throughout the body by the bloodstream, and it cannot be retrieved. Therefore, errors can be fatal. As shown in the following examples, the calculations are not difficult, but they are critical.

EXAMPLE PROBLEMS

1. You receive the following order to be prepared in the hospital pharmacy:

   Metoclopramide 12 mg in 50 mL D5W

   How many milliliters of metoclopramide (Reglan) injection with a concentration of 5 mg/mL would you need to prepare this solution?

$$12 \text{ mg} \times \frac{1 \text{ mL}}{5 \text{ mg}} = 2.4 \text{ mL}$$

2. You receive the following order for an IV infusion:

   Famotidine 25 mg in 100 mL of 5% dextrose

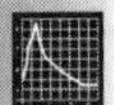

How many mL of famotidine (Pepcid) injection (10 mg/mL) should be used for this preparation?

$$25 \text{ mg} \times \frac{1 \text{ mL}}{10 \text{ mg}} = 2.5 \text{ mL}$$

3. A pharmacist gets the following physician's order:

Add 1 g of lidocaine to 250 mL IV solution

How much 2% lidocaine solution should be added?

$$2\% = 2 \text{ g}/100 \text{ mL}$$

$$1 \text{ g} \times \frac{100 \text{ mL}}{2 \text{ g}} = 50 \text{ mL}$$

4. The physician orders calcium gluceptate 540 mg to be added to IV fluids. You have available 5-mL ampules, each containing 90 mg of calcium gluceptate. How many milliliters would you add to the IV fluids to fill this order?

$$540 \text{ mg} \times \frac{5 \text{ mL}}{90 \text{ mg}} = 30 \text{ mL}$$

5. A patient is receiving D5½NS, and you receive an order to add 30 mEq of potassium chloride to the next 1-L bag of fluids. How much of a 14.9% KCl solution would you need to use?

(molecular weight of KCl = 74.5)

$$\frac{14.9 \text{ g}}{100 \text{ mL}} \times \frac{1{,}000 \text{ mg}}{1 \text{ g}} \times \frac{1 \text{ mEq}}{74.5 \text{ mg}} = 2 \text{ mEq/mL}$$

$$30 \text{ mEq} \times \frac{1 \text{ mL}}{2 \text{ mEq}} = 15 \text{ mL}$$

14.3 Flow Rate Calculations

The amount of drug administered via an IV solution depends on the flow rate of the solution.

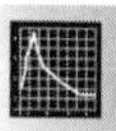

Definition. The *flow rate* of an IV solution is the volume administered over a period of time.

Expression. The flow rate is usually given as volume per time (i.e., mL/hr or mL/min) or drops per time based on the drop volume of the administration set used.

Discussion. The pharmacist must be able to calculate the flow rate for IV solutions. The flow rate may also be used to calculate the amount of drug delivered to a patient over a certain period of time or the length of time a certain volume of solution will last.

The concentration of the drug in the IV solution, the amount of drug to be administered to the patient, and the amount of time over which the drug should be infused will determine the flow rate for administration. The flow rate is usually rounded to the nearest whole number. Various nomograms are available for determining flow rate, in drops per minute, of an IV solution given the volume of solution, infusion time, and drop factor of the administration set. However, nomograms can be easily misread and should be used only to double-check a calculation.

Key Points. The flow rate of an IV solution is the final step in getting the correct amount of drug to the patient. This calculation is critical in delivering the proper dose, and a miscalculation can lead to improper dosing of the drug.

EXAMPLE PROBLEMS

1. A patient is to receive 1 L of 0.9% sodium chloride injection over 24 hours to keep his vein open in case IV medications need to be administered. What would be the flow rate (mL/hr) for this solution?

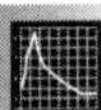

$$\frac{1\ \text{L}}{24\ \text{hr}} \times \frac{1{,}000\ \text{mL}}{1\ \text{L}} = 41.66\ \text{mL/hr} \approx 42\ \text{mL/hr}$$

2. A 1-L bag of lactated Ringer's injection is infused at a rate of 125 mL/hr. How long will the infusion last?

$$1\ \text{L} \times \frac{1{,}000\ \text{mL}}{1\ \text{L}} \times \frac{1\ \text{hr}}{125\ \text{mL}} = 8\ \text{hr}$$

3. A patient receives a solution by IV infusion at a rate of 36 gtt/min. How much solution is infused in 3 hours if the infusion set has a drop factor of 15 gtt/mL?

$$\frac{36\ \text{gtt}}{1\ \text{min}} \times \frac{60\ \text{min}}{1\ \text{hr}} \times 3\ \text{hr} \times \frac{1\ \text{mL}}{15\ \text{gtt}} = 432\ \text{mL}$$

4. The physician ordered 20 g of magnesium sulfate to be added to 1,000 mL D5W, and infused at 1.5 g/hr. What is the flow rate in mL/hr? (Assume negligible volume displacement by the $MgSO_4$.)

$$\frac{1.5\ \text{g}}{1\ \text{hr}} \times \frac{1{,}000\ \text{mL}}{20\ \text{g}} = 75\ \text{mL/hr}$$

5. At what flow rate (gtt/min) should the IV solution in Example Problem 4 infuse if the drop factor is 15 gtt/mL?

$$\frac{75\ \text{mL}}{1\ \text{hr}} \times \frac{15\ \text{gtt}}{1\ \text{mL}} \times \frac{1\ \text{hr}}{60\ \text{min}}$$

$$= 18.75\ \text{gtt/min} \approx 19\ \text{gtt/min}$$

6. A child weighing 15 kg is to receive potassium chloride at a dose of 1 mEq/kg over 6 hours. The final concentration of the infusion should be 20 mEq/L.

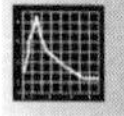

A. How many milliliters of an injection containing 2 mEq/mL should be used?

$$15 \text{ kg} \times \frac{1 \text{ mEq}}{1 \text{ kg}} = 15 \text{ mEq}$$

$$15 \text{ mEq} \times \frac{1 \text{ mL}}{2 \text{ mEq}} = 7.5 \text{ mL}$$

B. To what total volume should this dose be diluted with D5W?

$$15 \text{ mEq} \times \frac{1 \text{ L}}{20 \text{ mEq}} \times \frac{1{,}000 \text{ mL}}{1 \text{ L}} = 750 \text{ mL}$$

C. What should be the infusion rate in mL/min?

$$\frac{750 \text{ mL}}{6 \text{ hr}} \times \frac{1 \text{ hr}}{60 \text{ min}} = 2.08 \text{ mL/min} \approx 2 \text{ mL/min}$$

7. At 11:30 AM, you receive an order in the hospital pharmacy with instructions to decrease the flow rate on a patient's IV to 50 mL/hr. When you check this patient's profile, you find that he was receiving D5½NS 1,000 mL at 85 mL/hr and that the last bag was started at 9:00 AM. When should the next bag of D5½NS be started, assuming that the nurse changed the IV rate on the existing bag at 11:30 AM?

9:00 AM to 11:30 AM = 2.5 hr

$$\frac{85 \text{ mL}}{1 \text{ hr}} \times 2.5 \text{ hr} = 212.5 \text{ mL infused at 11:30 AM}$$

1,000 mL − 212.5 mL = 787.5 mL left at 11:30 AM

$$787.5 \text{ mL} \times \frac{1 \text{ hr}}{50 \text{ mL}} = 15.75 \text{ hr}$$

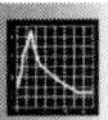

The IV will last for 15 hours, 45 minutes after the rate is changed to 50 mL/hr.

Adding 15 hours, 45 minutes to 11:30 AM, the next bag of IV solution should be started at 3:15 AM.

8. A patient whose body surface area is 1.5 m^2 is to receive 7.5 $mg/m^2/hr$ of cytarabine (Cytosar-U). How many drops/min of an IV infusion containing cytarabine 100 mg/L should be given, if the infusion set delivers 20 drops/mL?

$$\frac{7.5\ \text{mg}}{1\ \text{m}^2/\text{hr}} \times 1.5\ \text{m}^2 = 11.25\ \text{mg/hr}$$

$$\frac{11.25\ \text{mg}}{1\ \text{hr}} \times \frac{1\ \text{L}}{100\ \text{mg}} \times \frac{1{,}000\ \text{mL}}{1\ \text{L}} = 112.5\ \text{mL/hr}$$

$$\frac{112.5\ \text{mL}}{1\ \text{hr}} \times \frac{20\ \text{gtt}}{1\ \text{mL}} \times \frac{1\ \text{hr}}{60\ \text{min}} = 37.5\ \text{gtt/min} \approx 38\ \text{gtt/min}$$

9. A patient needs to receive 2 mg of bupivacaine (Marcaine) per day via an intrathecal pump. The concentration of bupivacaine in the pump reservoir is 0.25%, and the volume is 50 mL. What should be the infusion rate for this pump in mL/hr?

$$\frac{2\ \text{mg}}{1\ \text{day}} \times \frac{1\ \text{g}}{1{,}000\ \text{mg}} \times \frac{100\ \text{mL}}{0.25\ \text{g}} \times \frac{1\ \text{day}}{24\ \text{hr}} = 0.033\ \text{mL/hr}$$

10. A physician orders a 2-g vial of cephalothin sodium (Keflin) to be added to 500 mL of D5W. If the administration rate is 125 mL/hr, how many milligrams of cephalothin sodium will the patient receive per minute?

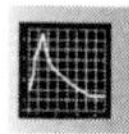

$$\frac{125\text{ mL}}{1\text{ hr}} \times \frac{1\text{ hr}}{60\text{ min}} \times \frac{2\text{ g}}{500\text{ mL}} \times \frac{1{,}000\text{ mg}}{1\text{ g}}$$
$$= 8.33\text{ mg/min}$$

11. The dose of imipenem-cilastatin (Primaxin) for a pediatric patient is 20 mg/kg q6h given intravenously over 30 minutes. A 250-mg vial is diluted to 100 mL using 0.9% NaCl and administered to a 24-lb child. What should be the flow rate in gtt/min if the infusion set delivers 60 gtt/mL?

$$\frac{20\text{ mg}}{1\text{ kg}} \times \frac{1\text{ kg}}{2.2\text{ lb}} \times 24\text{ lb} = 218.18\text{ mg}$$

$$\frac{218.18\text{ mg}}{30\text{ min}} \times \frac{100\text{ mL}}{250\text{ mg}} \times \frac{60\text{ gtt}}{1\text{ mL}}$$
$$= 174.55\text{ gtt/min} \approx 175\text{ gtt/min}$$

12. You receive a call in the hospital pharmacy at 4:30 AM informing you that the wrong IV solution was started on Mr. Jones, a diabetic patient. He was supposed to be receiving normal saline at 75 mL/hr and instead was given D5NS. The IV was started at 11:00 PM and has just been corrected. How much dextrose did this patient receive?

11:00 PM to 4:30 AM = 5.5 hr

$$\frac{75\text{ mL}}{1\text{ hr}} \times 5.5\text{ hr} = 412.5\text{ mL}$$

$$412.5\text{ mL} \times \frac{5\text{ g}}{100\text{ mL}} = 20.63\text{ g of dextrose}$$

13. If a solution containing 5% dextrose and 0.45% sodium chloride is infused at a rate of 60 mL/hr,

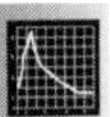

how many milliequivalents of sodium is the patient receiving per day?

$$\frac{60\ \text{mL}}{1\ \text{hr}} \times \frac{0.45\ \text{g}}{100\ \text{mL}} \times \frac{1{,}000\ \text{mg}}{1\ \text{g}} \times \frac{1\ \text{mEq}}{58.5\ \text{mg}} \times \frac{24\ \text{hr}}{1\ \text{day}} = 110.77\ \text{mEq/day}$$

14. You receive an order for amrinone lactate (Inocor) 250 mg/100 mL NS. This is to be administered to a 173-lb patient at a rate of 7.5 μg/kg/min. What would be the flow rate for this IV in mL/hr?

$$\frac{7.5\ \mu\text{g}}{1\ \text{kg/min}} \times \frac{1\ \text{kg}}{2.2\ \text{lb}} \times 173\ \text{lb} = 589.77\ \mu\text{g/min}$$

$$\frac{589.77\ \mu\text{g}}{1\ \text{min}} \times \frac{1\ \text{mg}}{1{,}000\ \mu\text{g}} \times \frac{100\ \text{mL}}{250\ \text{mg}} \times \frac{60\ \text{min}}{1\ \text{hr}} = 14.15\ \text{mL/hr} \approx 14\ \text{mL/hr}$$

15 NUTRITIONAL DOSING

Proper nutritional support is essential to aiding a patient in improving his or her disease status, and the caloric requirements for patients vary depending on their physical state and medical condition. The pharmacist must consider the caloric needs of a patient to supply the appropriate enteral or parenteral nutritional support. The purpose of this chapter is to assist the pharmacist with calculating the amounts of nutrients needed in parenteral or enteral therapy. Discussion of clinical assessment to determine nutritional needs of a patient is outside the scope of this chapter, and the reader should refer to a clinical therapeutics textbook for more information.

15.1 Determination of Nutritional Requirements

Nutrient requirements for a patient depend on his or her age, weight, height, and gender, as well as the patient's clinical condition, including disease state, nutrition status, and level of physical activity.

Definition. *Nutritional requirements* for a patient are the amounts of macronutrients (proteins, lipids, and carbohydrates) and micronutrients (vitamins, minerals, and electrolytes) needed to maintain or achieve a desired weight and health status.

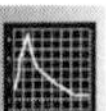

Expressions. The amounts of nutrients to fulfill a patient's requirements are usually expressed in weight units such as grams or milligrams. The amounts of electrolytes to be administered parenterally may be expressed in milliequivalents or millimoles.

Discussion. The steps in determining a patient's nutritional needs are as follows:

1. Calculate the total daily calories (TDC) using the Harris-Benedict equations and appropriate stress or activity factors (see Section 13.5).
2. Calculate the daily amount of amino acids (protein) required using 0.8 g per kilogram of body weight. This number may require adjustment for certain disease states as shown below:[1]

Renal dialysis	1.2 g/kg/day
Critical illness (e.g., sepsis or trauma)	1.5–2.0 g/kg/day
Severe burns	3.0 g/kg/day

3. Determine the number of calories supplied by the amino acids using the conversion 4 kcal supplied by 1 g of amino acids.
4. Calculate the amount of lipids needed by multiplying the TDC by 30% to 40%.[2] This calculation will give an answer in kilocalories, which must be converted to grams of lipids. Lipids, both enteral and parenteral, provide 9 kcal/g of energy. Lipids are administered parenterally as an emulsion, which uses carbohydrate-based emulsifying agents that also provide calories to the patient. The additional carbohydrate calories provided by the use of parenteral lipid emulsion can be accounted for by adding the carbohydrate calories to those provided by the lipid (9 kcal/g) component of the emulsion. Thus, if 20%

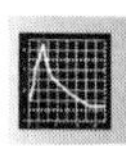

or 30% lipid emulsion is used to supply the lipids, 10 kcal/g of total energy is provided. If 10% lipid emulsion is used, 11 kcal/g of total energy is provided because of differences in the carbohydrate composition of the emulsions.[3]

5. Subtract the amount of calories contributed by lipids and amino acids from the TDC. There is some controversy regarding whether or not protein calories should be included in the overall caloric needs of the patient because amino acids are used for protein synthesis rather than as an energy source.[4] Therefore, the protein calories may be included or excluded as the pharmacist sees fit.
6. Calculate the amount of carbohydrate needed to contribute the remaining calories using the conversion factor of 4 kcal/g for enteral carbohydrates or 3.4 kcal/g for parenteral dextrose.

Once the amount of each nutrient has been calculated, the volume and type of solutions needed can be determined. Furthermore, the patient should also receive the recommended dietary allowances or dietary reference intakes of vitamins, minerals, and electrolytes.

To determine a patient's fluid requirements, the conversion used is 30 mL/kg of body weight or 1 mL/kcal of nutrition provided.[1] This value should be increased for patients who are dehydrated because of such conditions as vomiting and diarrhea, and decreased for patients who are experiencing renal failure or congestive heart failure.

Key Points. The calculations presented in this section are a beginning point for determining nutritional requirements; the patient must be monitored to ensure that adequate nutrition is being delivered.

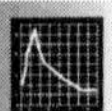

EXAMPLE PROBLEMS

1. The daily caloric requirement for a 58-year-old female who is 5′3″ tall and weighs 140 lb is 1,281.35 kcal/day according to the Harris-Benedict equation. Calculate the parenteral nutrition and fluid requirements for this patient, assuming that she has no disease states that would alter her nutritional requirements.

Protein:

$$140 \text{ lb} \times \frac{1 \text{ kg}}{2.2 \text{ lb}} \times \frac{0.8 \text{ g}}{1 \text{ kg/day}} = 50.91 \text{ g/day}$$

$$\frac{50.91 \text{ g}}{1 \text{ day}} \times \frac{4 \text{ kcal}}{1 \text{ g}} = 203.64 \text{ kcal/day}$$

Using an average lipid requirement of 35% of TDC and assuming that 10% lipid emulsion will be used:

$$1{,}281.35 \text{ kcal/day} \times 35\% = 448.47 \text{ kcal/day from lipid emulsion}$$

Lipids:

$$\frac{448.47 \text{ kcal}}{1 \text{ day}} \times \frac{1 \text{ g}}{11 \text{ kcal}} = 40.77 \text{ g/day}$$

$$1{,}281.35 \text{ kcal/day} - 203.64 \text{ kcal/day} - 448.47 \text{ kcal/day} = 629.24 \text{ kcal/day}$$

Dextrose:

$$\frac{629.24 \text{ kcal}}{1 \text{ day}} \times \frac{1 \text{ g}}{3.4 \text{ kcal}} = 185.07 \text{ g/day}$$

Fluid:

$$140 \text{ lb} \times \frac{1 \text{ kg}}{2.2 \text{ lb}} \times \frac{30 \text{ mL}}{1 \text{ kg/day}} = 1{,}909.09 \text{ mL/day}$$

Fluid: $$\frac{1{,}281.35 \text{ kcal}}{1 \text{ day}} \times \frac{1 \text{ mL}}{1 \text{ kcal}} = 1{,}281.35 \text{ mL/day}$$

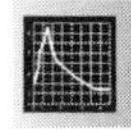

The patient should receive 50.91 g of protein, 40.77 g of lipids, 185.07 g of dextrose, and 1,281.35 to 1,909.09 mL of fluid per day.

2. The daily caloric requirement for a 76-year-old male who is 6′2″ tall and weighs 201 lb is 2,088.82 kcal/day. Calculate the enteral nutrition and fluid requirements for this patient, assuming that he has no disease states that would alter his nutritional requirements.

Protein: $201 \text{ lb} \times \frac{1 \text{ kg}}{2.2 \text{ lb}} \times \frac{0.8 \text{ g}}{1 \text{ kg/day}} = 73.09 \text{ g/day}$

$$\frac{73.09 \text{ g}}{1 \text{ day}} \times \frac{4 \text{ kcal}}{1 \text{ g}} = 292.36 \text{ kcal/day}$$

Using an average lipid requirement of 35% of TDC:

$$2{,}088.82 \text{ kcal/day} \times 35\% = 731.09 \text{ kcal/day}$$

Lipids: $\frac{731.09 \text{ kcal}}{1 \text{ day}} \times \frac{1 \text{ g}}{9 \text{ kcal}} = 81.23 \text{ g/day}$

$$2{,}088.82 \text{ kcal/day} - 292.36 \text{ kcal/day} - 731.09 \text{ kcal/day} = 1{,}065.37 \text{ kcal/day}$$

Carbohydrates:

$$\frac{1{,}065.37 \text{ kcal}}{1 \text{ day}} \times \frac{1 \text{ g}}{4 \text{ kcal}} = 266.34 \text{ g/day}$$

Fluid:

$$201 \text{ lb} \times \frac{1 \text{ kg}}{2.2 \text{ lb}} \times \frac{30 \text{ mL}}{1 \text{ kg/day}} = 2{,}740.91 \text{ mL/day}$$

Fluid:

$$\frac{2{,}088.82 \text{ kcal}}{1 \text{ day}} \times \frac{1 \text{ mL}}{1 \text{ kcal}} = 2{,}088.82 \text{ mL/day}$$

The patient should receive 73.09 g of protein, 81.23 g of lipids, 266.34 g of carbohydrates, and 2,088.82 to 2,740.91 mL of fluid per day.

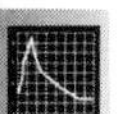

3. The daily caloric requirement for a 28-year-old female who is 5′5″ tall, weighs 132 lb, and is experiencing a severe infection is 2,513.84 kcal/day according to the Harris-Benedict equation and using an average stress factor of 1.8. Calculate the parenteral nutrition and fluid requirements for this patient, who has a severe infection.

Using an average protein requirement of 1.75 g/kg/day for a critically ill patient:

Protein: $132 \text{ lb} \times \dfrac{1 \text{ kg}}{2.2 \text{ lb}} \times \dfrac{1.75 \text{ g}}{1 \text{ kg/day}} = 105 \text{ g/day}$

$$\frac{105 \text{ g}}{1 \text{ day}} \times \frac{4 \text{ kcal}}{1 \text{ g}} = 420 \text{ kcal/day}$$

Using an average lipid requirement of 35% of TDC and assuming that a 20% lipid emulsion will be used:

$$2{,}513.84 \text{ kcal/day} \times 35\% = 879.85 \text{ kcal/day from lipid emulsion}$$

Lipids: $\dfrac{879.85 \text{ kcal}}{1 \text{ day}} \times \dfrac{1 \text{ g}}{10 \text{ kcal}} = 87.98 \text{ g/day}$

$$2{,}513.84 \text{ kcal/day} - 420 \text{ kcal/day} - 879.85 \text{ kcal/day} = 1{,}214 \text{ kcal/day}$$

Dextrose: $\dfrac{1{,}214 \text{ kcal}}{1 \text{ day}} \times \dfrac{1 \text{ g}}{3.4 \text{ kcal}} = 357.06 \text{ g/day}$

Fluid: $132 \text{ lb} \times \dfrac{1 \text{ kg}}{2.2 \text{ lb}} \times \dfrac{30 \text{ mL}}{1 \text{ kg/day}} = 1{,}800 \text{ mL/day}$

Fluid: $\dfrac{2{,}513.84 \text{ kcal}}{1 \text{ day}} \times \dfrac{1 \text{ mL}}{1 \text{ kcal}} = 2{,}513.84 \text{ mL/day}$

The patient should receive 105 g of protein, 87.98 g of lipids, 357.06 g of dextrose, and 1,800 to 2,513.84 mL of fluid per day.

15.2 Enteral Nutrition

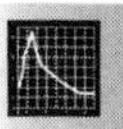

Enteral nutrition is preferred over parenteral nutrition if the patient's gastrointestinal tract is functioning properly due to lower cost and fewer complications. Furthermore, enteral nutrition maintains the structure and function of the gastrointestinal tract because it is not bypassed as in parenteral nutritional therapy.

Definition. *Enteral nutrition* is delivery of required nutrients via the gastrointestinal tract, including oral ingestion of food and delivery of liquid formulations by a tube. Usually, the term enteral nutrition is used to refer to the latter and is also used interchangeably with the term "tube feeding."

Expressions. Enteral nutrition usually includes a volume of formula to be administered, usually expressed in milliliters, and a flow rate at which to deliver the formula, usually expressed in milliliters per hour.

Discussion. Types of enteral formulas include polymeric, which consists of complex nutrients and is used only for patients with a fully functional gastrointestinal tract; monomeric and oligomeric, which consist of elemental nutrients and require less digestive capacity of the gastrointestinal tract; specialized, which is specially formulated for specific diseases such as renal or hepatic failure; and modular, which consists of separate protein, carbohydrate, and fat formulas that can be combined to prepare patient-specific formulas or to supplement commercially available formulas. With more than 100 enteral formulas available on the market, selection of the proper formula for a patient can be quite complicated. Factors to consider in selecting the proper formula include patient characteristics such as gastrointestinal

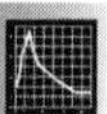

tract functionality, disease status, and nutritional needs and characteristics of the formula such as caloric density, osmolality, percent free water, and relative amounts of the various nutrients.

Administration methods for enteral nutrition include continuous, in which the formula is delivered over 16 to 24 hours daily; continuous cyclic, in which the formula is delivered over 10 to 14 hours daily; intermittent, in which 240 to 480 mL of formula is infused over 20 to 40 minutes four to six times daily; and bolus feeding, in which 240 to 480 mL of formula is delivered over less than 10 minutes four to six times daily.[5] The delivery method depends on the anatomic location of the feeding tube, condition of the patient, and the patient's environment (e.g., formula administered in the hospital or at home).

Pharmacy Applications. In many cases, the pharmacist may work in conjunction with a dietician or other health care provider to select and monitor an enteral nutrition regimen for a patient.

EXAMPLE PROBLEMS

1. The nutritional requirements for a 76-year-old male who is 6′2″ tall and weighs 201 lb are as follows: (see Example Problem 2 in Section 15.1)

Protein:	73.09 g/day
Lipids:	81.23 g/day
Carbohydrates:	266.34 g/day
Water:	2,088.82–2,740.91 mL/day
Total calories:	2,088.82 kcal/day

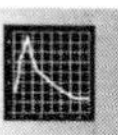

Ensure liquid is chosen for enteral therapy for this patient, and a 1-quart container provides 37 g protein, 143 g carbohydrates, and 37 g lipids, and has an osmolality of 470 mOsmol/kg and a caloric density of 1.06 kcal/mL.[6]

A. Based on the total calories needed per day, how much Ensure should this patient receive?

$$\frac{2{,}088.82 \text{ kcal}}{1 \text{ day}} \times \frac{1 \text{ mL}}{1.06 \text{ kcal}} = 1{,}970.58 \text{ mL/day}$$

B. How much of each nutrient would this volume of Ensure deliver per day?

Protein:

$$\frac{1{,}970.58 \text{ mL}}{1 \text{ day}} \times \frac{1 \text{ qt}}{946 \text{ mL}} \times \frac{37 \text{ g}}{1 \text{ qt}} = 77.07 \text{ g/day}$$

Carbohydrates:

$$\frac{1{,}970.58 \text{ mL}}{1 \text{ day}} \times \frac{1 \text{ qt}}{946 \text{ mL}} \times \frac{143 \text{ g}}{1 \text{ qt}} = 297.88 \text{ g/day}$$

Lipids:

$$\frac{1{,}970.58 \text{ mL}}{1 \text{ day}} \times \frac{1 \text{ qt}}{946 \text{ mL}} \times \frac{37 \text{ g}}{1 \text{ qt}} = 77.07 \text{ g/day}$$

C. Does this regimen meet the patient's water requirements?

Enteral formulas with a caloric density of 1 to 1.2 kcal/day usually contain 80% to 85% free water.[7]

1,970.58 mL/day × 80% = 1,576.47 mL/day

1,970.58 mL/day × 85% = 1,675 mL/day

Therefore, the amount of water provided by 1,970.58 mL of formula would be 1,576.47 to

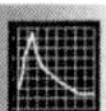

1,675 mL/day. The amount of water delivered falls short of the amount required by the patient by 413.82 to 1,164.44 mL. The amount of water used to flush the feeding tube may be sufficient to meet the additional water needs, but the patient should be monitored for signs of dehydration.

D. If the formula is to be delivered continuously over a 24-hour period, what would be the flow rate in mL/hr?

$$\frac{1{,}970.58 \text{ mL}}{1 \text{ day}} \times \frac{1 \text{ day}}{24 \text{ hr}} = 82.11 \text{ mL/hr} \approx 82 \text{ mL/hr}$$

E. If the patient is to continue receiving this formula at home by intermittent feedings over 40 minutes every 4 hours, what volume would be administered with each feeding, and what would be the flow rate in mL/hr?

$$\frac{1{,}970.58 \text{ mL}}{1 \text{ day}} \times \frac{1 \text{ day}}{24 \text{ hr}} \times \frac{4 \text{ hr}}{1 \text{ dose}} = 328.43 \text{ mL/dose}$$

$$\frac{328.43 \text{ mL}}{40 \text{ min}} \times \frac{60 \text{ min}}{1 \text{ hr}} = 492.65 \text{ mL/hr} \approx 493 \text{ mL/hr}$$

2. A mother discusses with her pharmacist that each day she has been giving her son three 237-mL containers of Resource Just for Kids chocolate-flavored formula to “keep him healthy because he doesn’t eat much.”

A. How much formula is the child consuming each day?

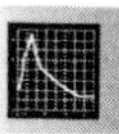

$$\frac{237 \text{ mL}}{1 \text{ container}} \times \frac{3 \text{ containers}}{1 \text{ day}} = 711 \text{ mL/day}$$

B. Resource Just for Kids supplies 30 g of protein, 110 g of carbohydrates, and 50 g of lipids per liter of formula, and has a caloric density of 1 kcal/mL.[6] How much of each nutrient and how many calories is the child receiving from this formula each day?

Protein:

$$\frac{30 \text{ g}}{1 \text{ L}} \times \frac{1 \text{ L}}{1{,}000 \text{ mL}} \times \frac{711 \text{ mL}}{1 \text{ day}} = 21.33 \text{ g/day}$$

Carbohydrates:

$$\frac{110 \text{ g}}{1 \text{ L}} \times \frac{1 \text{ L}}{1{,}000 \text{ mL}} \times \frac{711 \text{ mL}}{1 \text{ day}} = 78.21 \text{ g/day}$$

Lipids:

$$\frac{50 \text{ g}}{1 \text{ L}} \times \frac{1 \text{ L}}{1{,}000 \text{ mL}} \times \frac{711 \text{ mL}}{1 \text{ day}} = 35.55 \text{ g/day}$$

Total calories: $\frac{711 \text{ mL}}{1 \text{ day}} \times \frac{1 \text{ kcal}}{1 \text{ mL}} = 711 \text{ kcal/day}$

C. Resource Just for Kids also supplies 380 mg of sodium and 1,300 mg of potassium per liter.[6] How many milliequivalents of sodium and potassium is the child receiving per day? (molecular weight of Na = 23, molecular weight of K = 39)

Sodium:

$$\frac{380 \text{ mg}}{1 \text{ L}} \times \frac{1 \text{ mEq}}{23 \text{ mg}} \times \frac{1 \text{ L}}{1{,}000 \text{ mL}} \times \frac{711 \text{ mL}}{1 \text{ day}} = 11.75 \text{ mEq/day}$$

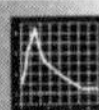

Potassium:

$$\frac{1{,}300 \text{ mg}}{1 \text{ L}} \times \frac{1 \text{ mEq}}{39 \text{ mg}} \times \frac{1 \text{ L}}{1{,}000 \text{ mL}} \times \frac{711 \text{ mL}}{1 \text{ day}} = 23.7 \text{ mEq/day}$$

15.3 Parenteral Nutrition

Parenteral nutrition is used for patients who cannot ingest or absorb nutrients via the gastrointestinal tract. Total parenteral nutrition supplies all required nutrients, and partial parenteral nutrition supplements the patient's nutritional needs when adequate calories or nutrients cannot be administered enterally.

Definition. *Parenteral nutrition* is the delivery of required nutrients by a parenteral route, usually intravenously. Parenteral nutrition solutions are also called TPNs, which stands for total parenteral nutrition, or hyperals, which stands for hyperalimentation solutions.

Expressions. Parenteral nutrition usually includes a volume of solution to be administered, usually expressed in milliliters, and a flow rate at which to deliver the solution, usually expressed in milliliters per hour.

Discussion. Parenteral nutrition differs from enteral nutrition in that the solutions administered are usually patient-specific. Calculated volumes of amino acid and dextrose solutions and lipid emulsions are used to prepare intravenous admixtures to provide the required nutrients for the patient. The concentration of these solutions and emulsions is usually expressed as percent

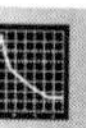

weight-in-volume (see Section 4.1). In addition to nutrients, these parenteral nutrition solutions usually also contain electrolytes with amounts expressed as milliequivalents (see Section 10.1), as well as vitamins and minerals. This mixture may be administered via a central or peripheral vein, depending on the osmolarity (see Section 10.3), and at a continuous or intermittent flow rate depending on the needs of the patient.

EXAMPLE PROBLEMS

1. The nutritional requirements for a 58-year-old female who is 5′3″ tall and weighs 140 lb are as follows (see Example Problem 1 in Section 15.1):

Amino acids:	50.91 g/day
Lipids:	40.77 g/day
Dextrose:	185.07 g/day
Fluids:	1,281.35–1,909.09 mL/day
Total calories:	1,281.35 kcal/day

A. How much 7% amino acid solution, 10% lipid emulsion, and 50% dextrose solution should be used to administer the required nutrients?

Amino acids:

$$\frac{50.91\text{ g}}{1\text{ day}} \times \frac{100\text{ mL}}{7\text{ g}} \times 727.27\text{ mL/day}$$

Lipids: $\dfrac{40.77\text{ g}}{1\text{ day}} \times \dfrac{100\text{ mL}}{10\text{ g}} = 407.7\text{ mL/day}$

Dextrose:

$$\frac{185.07\text{ g}}{1\text{ day}} \times \frac{100\text{ mL}}{50\text{ g}} = 370.14\text{ mL/day}$$

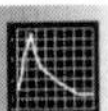

B. What would be the total volume of this mixture, and will it meet the patient's fluid requirement?

$$727.27 \text{ mL/day} + 407.7 \text{ mL/day} + 370.14 \text{ mL/day} = 1{,}505.11 \text{ mL/day}$$

The volume of 1,505.11 mL meets the patient's fluid requirement.

C. What would be the flow rate of this solution in mL/hr?

$$\frac{1{,}505.11 \text{ mL}}{1 \text{ day}} \times \frac{1 \text{ day}}{24 \text{ hr}} = 62.71 \text{ mL/hr} \approx 63 \text{ mL/hr}$$

2. The nutritional requirements for a 28-year-old female who is 5′5″ tall, weighs 132 lb, and is experiencing a severe infection are as follows (see Example Problem 3 in Section 15.1):

Amino acids:	105 g/day
Lipids:	87.98 g/day
Dextrose:	357.06 g/day
Fluids:	1,800–2,513.84 mL/day
Total calories:	2,513.84 kcal/day

A. How much 15% amino acid solution, 20% lipid emulsion, and 70% dextrose solution should be used to administer the required nutrients?

$$\text{Amino acids: } \frac{105 \text{ g}}{1 \text{ day}} \times \frac{100 \text{ mL}}{15 \text{ g}} = 700 \text{ mL/day}$$

$$\text{Lipids: } \frac{87.98 \text{ g}}{1 \text{ day}} \times \frac{100 \text{ mL}}{20 \text{ g}} = 439.92 \text{ mL/day}$$

Dextrose:

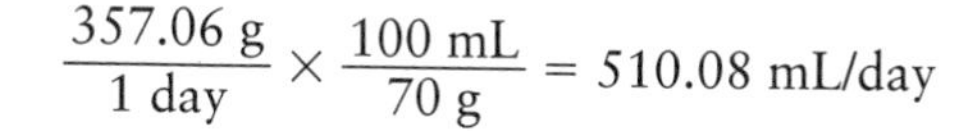

$$\frac{357.06\ \text{g}}{1\ \text{day}} \times \frac{100\ \text{mL}}{70\ \text{g}} = 510.08\ \text{mL/day}$$

B. What would be the total volume of this mixture, and will it meet the patient's fluid requirement?

$$700\ \text{mL/day} + 439.92\ \text{mL/day} + 510.08\ \text{mL/day} = 1{,}650\ \text{mL/day}$$

The volume of 1,650 mL does not meet the patient's fluid requirement; therefore, a minimum of approximately 150 mL of additional sterile water for injection should be added to each daily TPN solution to ensure adequate hydration.

C. Because the patient has a severe infection and is probably running a fever, the pharmacist decides to add enough sterile water for injection to reach a final volume of 2,000 mL. What would be the flow rate of this solution in mL/hr?

$$\frac{2{,}000\ \text{mL}}{1\ \text{day}} \times \frac{1\ \text{day}}{24\ \text{hr}} = 83.33\ \text{mL/hr} \approx 83\ \text{mL/hr}$$

D. What would be the percentage strength of amino acids, dextrose, and lipids in the TPN solution after dilution to 2,000 mL?

Amino acids: $\frac{105\ \text{g}}{2{,}000\ \text{mL}} \times 100 = 5.25\%$

Lipids: $\frac{87.98\ \text{g}}{2{,}000\ \text{mL}} \times 100 = 4.4\%$

Dextrose: $\frac{357.06\ \text{g}}{2{,}000\ \text{mL}} \times 100 = 17.85\%$

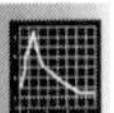

3. A pharmacist receives the following order for a parenteral nutrition solution:

		Strength Commercially Available
Amino acids 8.5%	500 mL	8.5% w/v
Dextrose 50%	500 mL	50% w/v
Sodium chloride	25 mEq	4 mEq/mL
Potassium chloride	20 mEq	2 mEq/mL
Magnesium sulfate	8 mEq	4.08 mEq/mL
Calcium gluconate	10 mEq	0.465 mEq/mL
Potassium phosphate	21 mmol	3 mmol/mL
MVI-12	10 mL	10-mL vial
Trace elements	3 mL	3-mL vial

A. Calculate the volume of each additive needed and the final volume of the solution.

Amino acids 8.5%: 500 mL

Dextrose 50%: 500 mL

Sodium chloride: $25 \text{ mEq} \times \dfrac{1 \text{ mL}}{4 \text{ mEq}} = 6.25 \text{ mL}$

Potassium chloride: $20 \text{ mEq} \times \dfrac{1 \text{ mL}}{2 \text{ mEq}} = 10 \text{ mL}$

Magnesium sulfate: $8 \text{ mEq} \times \dfrac{1\text{mL}}{4.08 \text{ mEq}} = 1.96 \text{ mL}$

Calcium gluconate: $10 \text{ mEq} \times \dfrac{1 \text{ mL}}{0.465 \text{ mEq}} = 21.51 \text{ mL}$

Potassium phosphate: $21 \text{ mmol} \times \frac{1 \text{ mL}}{3 \text{ mmol}} = 7 \text{ mL}$

MVI-12: 10 mL

Trace elements: 3 mL

Total volume = 1,059.72 mL

B. How many kcal/day would the patient receive if the flow rate for the TPN were 75 mL/hr?

Amino acids:

$$\frac{8.5 \text{ g}}{100 \text{ mL}} \times 500 \text{ mL} \times \frac{4 \text{ kcal}}{1 \text{ g}} = 170 \text{ kcal}$$

Dextrose:

$$\frac{50 \text{ g}}{100 \text{ mL}} \times 500 \text{ mL} \times \frac{3.4 \text{ kcal}}{1 \text{ g}} = 850 \text{ kcal}$$

170 kcal + 850 kcal = 1,020 kcal in TPN

$$\frac{1{,}020 \text{ kcal}}{1{,}059.72 \text{ mL}} \times \frac{75 \text{ mL}}{1 \text{ hr}} \times \frac{24 \text{ hr}}{1 \text{ day}} = 1{,}732.53 \text{ kcal/day}$$

C. If the patient also receives 500 mL of a 10% lipid emulsion daily, how many total calories is he receiving per day?

$$\frac{10 \text{ g}}{100 \text{ mL}} \times \frac{500 \text{ mL}}{1 \text{ day}} \times \frac{11 \text{ kcal}}{1 \text{ g}} = 550 \text{ kcal/day}$$

$$550 \text{ kcal/day} + 1{,}732.53 \text{ kcal/day} = 2{,}282.53 \text{ kcal/day}$$

4. A pharmacist receives the following order for a parenteral nutrition solution:

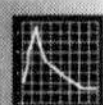

		Component Source
Amino acids	2.5%	500 mL of 6% amino acids injection
Dextrose	25%	500 mL of 70% dextrose injection
Sodium acetate	20 mEq	50-mL vial of 32.8% solution
Potassium chloride	15 mEq	25-mL vial of 14.9% solution
Magnesium sulfate	10 mEq	10-mL vial of 12.5% magnesium sulfate heptahydrate solution
Calcium chloride	5 mEq	50-mL vial of 10% solution
Potassium phosphate	15 mmol	10-mL vial of 3 mmol/mL solution
Water q.s.	1,000 mL	1,000 mL of sterile water for injection

What volume of each ingredient would be needed to prepare this solution?

Amino acids:

$$\frac{2.5\text{ g}}{100\text{ mL}} \times 1{,}000\text{ mL} \times \frac{100\text{ mL}}{6\text{ g}} = 416.67\text{ mL}$$

Dextrose:

$$\frac{25\text{ g}}{100\text{ mL}} \times 1{,}000\text{ mL} \times \frac{100\text{ mL}}{70\text{ g}} = 357.14\text{ mL}$$

Sodium acetate ($NaC_2H_3O_2$, molecular weight = 82):

$$20\text{ mEq} \times \frac{82\text{ mg}}{1\text{ mEq}} \times \frac{1\text{ g}}{1{,}000\text{ mg}} \times \frac{100\text{ mL}}{32.8\text{ g}} = 5\text{ mL}$$

Potassium chloride (KCl, molecular weight = 74.5):

$$15 \text{ mEq} \times \frac{74.5 \text{ mg}}{1 \text{ mEq}} \times \frac{1 \text{ g}}{1{,}000 \text{ mg}} \times \frac{100 \text{ mL}}{14.9 \text{ g}} = 7.5 \text{ mL}$$

Magnesium sulfate
($MgSO_4 \cdot 7H_2O$, molecular weight = 246):

$$10 \text{ mEq} \times \frac{246 \text{ mg}}{2 \text{ mEq}} \times \frac{1 \text{ g}}{1{,}000 \text{ mg}} \times \frac{100 \text{ mL}}{12.5 \text{ g}} = 9.84 \text{ mL}$$

Calcium chloride ($CaCl_2$, molecular weight = 111):

$$5 \text{ mEq} \times \frac{111 \text{ mg}}{2 \text{ mEq}} \times \frac{1 \text{ g}}{1{,}000 \text{ mg}} \times \frac{100 \text{ mL}}{10 \text{ g}} = 2.78 \text{ mL}$$

Potassium phosphate: $15 \text{ mmol} \times \frac{1 \text{ mL}}{3 \text{ mmol}} = 5 \text{ mL}$

NOTE: The concentration of the potassium phosphate injection is given in millimoles of phosphate per milliliter because the solution consists of a mixture of potassium phosphate, monobasic, and potassium phosphate, dibasic (see Example Problem 4 in Section 10.2).

Total volume = 803.93 mL

Amount of water to add:

$$1{,}000 \text{ mL} - 803.93 \text{ mL} = 196.07 \text{ mL}$$

References

1. Dipiro JT, Talbert RL, Yee GC, Matzke G, Wells BG, Posey LM, eds. Pharmacotherapy: A Pathophysiologic Approach. 5th Ed. New York, NY: McGraw-Hill, 2002:2456–2457, 2523.
2. Dipiro JT, Talbert RL, Yee GC, Matzke G, Wells BG, Posey LM, eds. Pharmacotherapy: A Pathophysiologic Approach. 5th Ed. New York, NY: McGraw-Hill, 2002:2485.

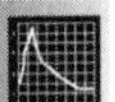

3. Dipiro JT, Talbert RL, Yee GC, Matzke G, Wells BG, Posey LM, eds. Pharmacotherapy: A Pathophysiologic Approach. 5th Ed. New York, NY: McGraw-Hill, 2002:2480.
4. Miles JM, Klein JA. Should protein be included in caloric calculations for a TPN prescription? Point-counterpoint. Nutrition in Clinical Practice 1996;11:204–206.
5. Dipiro JT, Talbert RL, Yee GC, Matzke G, Wells BG, Posey LM, eds. Pharmacotherapy: A Pathophysiologic Approach. 5th Ed. New York, NY: McGraw-Hill, 2002:2501–2502.
6. CliniSphere 2.0 [book on CD ROM]. St. Louis, MO: Facts and Comparisons, 2002.
7. Koda-Kimble MA, Young LY, eds. Applied Therapeutics: The Clinical Use of Drugs. 7th Ed. Baltimore, MD: Lippincott Williams & Wilkins, 2001:34–43.

16

VETERINARY DOSING

Veterinary medicine, like human medicine, uses pharmaceuticals of various dosage forms and strengths in the treatment of disease and illness. Because animals suffer from many of the same conditions afflicting humans, such as infectious disease, cardiovascular disease, cancer, etc., many of the medications used in human medicine are also used in animal medicine. Other drugs are developed for diseases that are specific to animal species.[1–2]

Pharmacists often are called on to fill the prescription orders of veterinarians. It should be noted that the abbreviation "sid," meaning "once per day," is commonly used in veterinary prescriptions.

Discussion. The dosage forms used in veterinary medicine are the same types as those used in human medicine. However, specialized drug-delivery devices commonly are used to administer the dosage forms, including esophageal, mastitis, and pole-mounted syringes, drench guns, and oral tubes designed to deliver medication directly into an animal's stomach.[3]

Veterinary patients range from birds, fish, and small domestic pets to various farm animals, thoroughbred horses, and exotic animal species of the jungle or zoological park. Consequently, the magnitude of doses varies widely. In addition to animal size, consideration of species is important, because each species represents

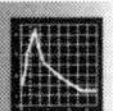

unique physiologic and pharmacokinetic characteristics. Readers are referred to standard texts in veterinary medicine regarding this aspect of animal dosing.[1–2]

Key Points. The calculation of animal dosage generally is based on an animal's weight or body surface area (BSA). Although the *methods* of such dosage calculations are the same for human and veterinary patients, there are substantial differences in drug dosage levels and in the calculation of BSA, as shown by Table 16-1 for the calculation of the BSA for dogs and cats.

16.1 Based on Body Weight

Veterinary dosing based on weight is an especially important factor. Consider this contrast: a pet cockatiel may weigh less than 100 g; a cat, several pounds; a race horse, 1,000 lb; and an elephant, 12,000 lb or more. Even among pet dogs, the range is dramatic, from the small "toy" dogs such as the Chihuahua, which may weigh 2 lb, to the Saint Bernard, which may weigh up to 180 lb.

EXAMPLE PROBLEMS

1. Allopurinol may be administered to parakeets for gout by crushing one 100-mg tablet, adding water to 10 mL, and administering 1 drop qid. Using a dropper that delivers 20 drops/mL, calculate the milligrams of allopurinol administered daily.

$$\frac{100 \text{ mg}}{10 \text{ mL}} \times \frac{1 \text{ mL}}{20 \text{ drops}} \times \frac{1 \text{ drop}}{\text{dose}} \times 4 \text{ doses} = 2 \text{ mg}$$

2. Furosemide is used in the treatment of CHF in animals at a maintenance dose of 0.5 mg/kg sid. Calculate the dose for a 15-lb dog.

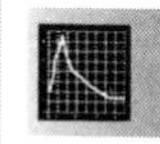

TABLE 16-1

Weight to Body Surface Area Conversion for Dogs and Cats

BSA in square meters = K × (body weight in grams$^{2/3}$) × 10^{-4}
K = constant (10.1 for dogs and 10.0 for cats)

Dogs		Dogs		Cats	
Body wt (kg)	BSA (m^2)	Body wt (kg)	BSA (m^2)	Body wt (kg)	BSA (m^2)
0.5	0.06	26	0.88	0.5	0.06
1	0.10	27	0.90	1	0.10
2	0.15	28	0.92	1.5	0.12
3	0.20	29	0.94	2	0.15
4	0.25	30	0.96	2.5	0.17
5	0.29	31	0.99	3	0.20
6	0.33	32	1.01	3.5	0.22
7	0.36	33	1.03	4	0.24
8	0.40	34	1.05	4.5	0.26
9	0.43	35	1.07	5	0.28
10	0.46	36	1.09	5.5	0.29
11	0.49	37	1.11	6	0.31
12	0.52	38	1.13	6.5	0.33
13	0.55	39	1.15	7	0.34
14	0.58	40	1.17	7.5	0.36
15	0.60	41	1.19	8	0.38
16	0.63	42	1.21	8.5	0.39
17	0.66	43	1.23	9	0.41
18	0.69	44	1.25	9.5	0.42
19	0.71	45	1.26	10	0.44
20	0.74	46	1.28		
21	0.76	47	1.30		
22	0.78	48	1.32		
23	0.81	49	1.34		
24	0.83	50	1.36		
25	0.85				

Adapted with permission from Rosenthal RC. Chemotherapy. In: Ettinger SJ, Feldman EC, Eds. Textbook of Internal Medicine, Diseases of the Dog and Cat. 4th Ed. Philadelphia, PA: W.B. Saunders Company, 1995.

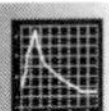

$$\frac{0.5\text{ mg}}{1\text{ kg}} \times \frac{1\text{ kg}}{2.2\text{ lb}} \times 15\text{ lb} = 3.4\text{ mg}$$

3. A cockatiel may be given 6 mg of ketamine intramuscularly for anesthesia. Calculate the dose, on a mg/kg basis, for an 85-g cockatiel.

$$\frac{6\text{ mg}}{85\text{ g}} \times \frac{1{,}000\text{ g}}{1\text{ kg}} = 70.6\text{ mg/kg}$$

4. Acetazolamide may be used as adjunct therapy for glaucoma in cats at a dose of 7 mg/kg. Acetazolamide is available in 125-mg tablets. If one tablet is crushed and mixed into 30 g of cat food, what weight of the food would contain a dose of medication for an 11-lb cat?

$$\frac{7\text{ mg}}{1\text{ kg}} \times \frac{1\text{ kg}}{2.2\text{ lb}} \times \frac{30\text{ g food}}{125\text{ mg}} \times 11\text{ lb} = 8.4\text{ g food}$$

5. Albuterol sulfate is administered orally to horses for bronchospasm at a dose of 8 μg/kg. Calculate the number of milliliters of an 0.083% solution of albuterol sulfate to administer to a 900-lb horse.

$$\frac{8\ \mu\text{g}}{1\text{ kg}} \times \frac{1\text{ kg}}{2.2\text{ lb}} \times 900\text{ lb} = 3{,}272.73\ \mu\text{g}$$

$$\frac{100\text{ mL}}{0.083\text{ g}} \times \frac{1\text{ g}}{1{,}000{,}000\ \mu\text{g}} \times 3{,}272.73\ \mu\text{g} = 3.94\text{ mL}$$

16.2 Based on Body Surface Area

An animal's BSA may be used in determining drug dosage. Specialized tables for determining the BSA for small animals have been developed.[4]

EXAMPLE PROBLEMS

Note: Table 16-1 is used in solving the following problems.

1. The dose of methotrexate sodium for neoplastic disease in cats is 2.5 mg/m^2 po twice weekly. Calculate the single dose for a 2-kg cat.

2-kg cat = 0.15 m^2 BSA

$$\frac{2.5\ \text{mg}}{\text{m}^2} \times 0.15\ \text{m}^2 = 0.375\ \text{mg}$$

2. Medetomide hydrochloride may be used as a sedative in dogs at a dose of 750 µg/m^2. How many milliliters of a solution containing 1 mg of drug/mL should be administered to a 10-kg dog?

10-kg dog = 0.46 m^2 BSA

$$\frac{750\ \mu\text{g}}{\text{m}^2} \times \frac{1\ \text{mL}}{1\ \text{mg}} \times \frac{1\ \text{mg}}{1{,}000\ \mu\text{g}} \times 0.46\ \text{m}^2 = 0.345\ \text{mL}$$

3. The maximum dose of doxorubicin in canine chemotherapy is 200 mg/m^2. Calculate the maximum dose for a dog weighing 20 kg.

20-kg dog = 0.74 m^2 BSA

$$\frac{200\ \text{mg}}{\text{m}^2} \times 0.74\ \text{m}^2 = 148\ \text{mg}$$

4. For large breed dogs, the dose of digoxin is 0.22 mg/m^2. Calculate the dose for a dog weighing 22 kg.

22-kg dog = 0.78 m^2 BSA

$$\frac{0.22\ \text{mg}}{\text{m}^2} \times 0.78\ \text{m}^2 = 0.17\ \text{mg}$$

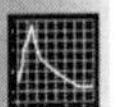

References

1. Aiello S, ed. The Merck Veterinary Manual. 8th Ed. Whitehouse Station, NJ: Merck & Co, 1998.
2. Plumb DC. Veterinary Drug Handbook. 3rd Ed. Ames, IA: Iowa State University Press, 1999.
3. Allen LV Jr, ed. Animal drug delivery systems. International Journal of Pharmaceutical Compounding 1997;1:229. Adapted from: Blodinger J. Formulation of Veterinary Dosage Forms. New York, NY: Marcel Dekker, 1983.
4. Rosenthal RC. Chemotherapy. In: Ettinger SJ, Feldman EC, eds. Textbook of Internal Medicine, Diseases of the Dog and Cat. 4th Ed. Philadelphia, PA: W.B. Saunders Company, 1995.

17

CONSIDERATION OF DRUGS REQUIRING PATIENT-SPECIFIC DOSING

The vast majority of drugs have a wide enough therapeutic window to accommodate interpatient variability. This variability, however, for some drugs significantly affects dosing guidelines, and specific doses must be calculated for each patient. Many of these individualized doses are based on pharmacokinetic parameters derived from patient data; therefore, the reader may need to refer to Chapter 12 for an overview of pharmacokinetics, or to a more comprehensive source. These calculations usually also require determination of patient parameters such as creatinine clearance (CrCl) and ideal body weight (IBW), which are presented in Chapter 13 on pages 172 and 166, respectively.

17.1 Aminoglycosides

Aminoglycoside antibiotics include gentamicin, tobramycin, netilmicin, amikacin, streptomycin, and kanamycin. The doses for these antibiotics must be individualized based on the patient's body weight, renal

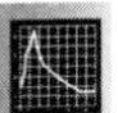

function, and measured serum concentrations of the drug to maintain therapeutic levels but avoid serious adverse reactions.

Discussion. The pharmacokinetic parameters and dosage regimen for aminoglycosides can be calculated as follows[1]:

1. Calculate the patient's creatinine clearance (CrCl) using the Cockcroft-Gault equation and IBW.
2. Calculate the elimination rate constant (k, in hours^{-1}) using the following equation:

$$k = 0.00293 \times CrCl + 0.014$$

3. In normal-weight patients, the volume of distribution (V_D, in liters) can be calculated as follows:

$$V_D = 0.26 \text{ L/kg} \times \text{Weight (in kg)}$$

If the patient's actual body weight is greater than 30% of IBW, the patient's excess adipose tissue can be taken into account using the following equation:

$$V_D = 0.26 \text{ L/kg} \times [IBW + 0.4(TBW - IBW)]$$

where TBW is the patient's total body weight or actual body weight.

4. Choose appropriate peak ($C_{max,ss}$) and trough ($C_{min,ss}$) serum values for the specific aminoglycoside from the following chart:[2]

Drug	Peak (μg/mL)	Trough (μg/mL)
Amikacin	16–32	1–8
Gentamicin	4–8	0.5–2
Kanamycin	15–40	5–10
Netilmicin	6–10	0.5–2
Streptomycin	20–30	<5
Tobramycin	4–8	0.5–2

Note that the units of concentration are in μg/mL. To obtain the desired units in the answer, the units of μg/mL are often used interchangeably with equivalent units of mg/L as shown below:

$$\frac{16\ \mu g}{1\ mL} \times \frac{1\ mg}{1{,}000\ \mu g} \times \frac{1{,}000\ mL}{1\ L} = 16\ mg/L$$

5. Calculate the dosing interval (τ, in hours) needed to achieve the concentrations chosen above using the following equation:

$$\tau = \frac{\ln C_{max,ss} - \ln C_{min,ss}}{k} + T$$

where T is the infusion time for the antibiotic solution.

The value calculated for τ is usually rounded off to an acceptable dosing interval (e.g., 8, 12, 24 hours).

6. Calculate the dose (D, in mg) using the following formula:

$$D = TkV_DC_{max,ss}\left(\frac{1 - e^{-k\tau}}{1 - e^{-kT}}\right)$$

This dose is then rounded off to the nearest 5 to 10 mg.

7. If a loading dose (LD) is needed, it can be calculated using the following equation:

$$LD = C_{max,ss} \times V_D$$

These calculations provide an initial dose and dosing interval for a patient. The patient should be evaluated and doses should be adjusted based on the measured serum levels of the drug. To adjust a patient's dose to achieve appropriate serum concentrations of the drug, whether or not the patient has reached steady-state should first

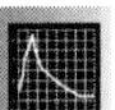

be established. The patient is approximately at steady-state after an estimated three to five half-lives have passed, and the half-life ($t_{1/2}$) can be calculated using the following equation:

$$t_{1/2} = \frac{0.693}{k}$$

where k is the elimination rate constant calculated in Step 2 above.

If the patient has not reached steady-state, a serum aminoglycoside concentration should be obtained:

- Before a dose (C_{min})
- After a 1-hour infusion of the drug or a 30-minute infusion followed by a 30-minute waiting time to allow for drug distribution (C_{max})
- Approximately one estimated half-life after C_{max} (C_3)

Using C_{max}, C_3, and the time elapsed between these measurements (Δt, in hours), the following calculation can be used to calculate a new elimination rate constant:

$$k = \frac{\ln C_{max} - \ln C_3}{\Delta t}$$

If the patient has reached steady-state, a serum aminoglycoside concentration should be obtained:

- Before a dose ($C_{min,ss}$)
- After a 1-hour infusion of the drug or a 30-minute infusion followed by a 30-minute waiting time to allow for drug distribution ($C_{max,ss}$)

Using these two concentrations, the dosage interval (τ, in hours), and the infusion time or infusion time plus waiting time (T, in hours), the following calculation can be used to calculate a new elimination rate constant:

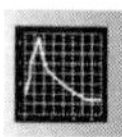

$$k = \frac{\ln C_{max,ss} - \ln C_{min,ss}}{\tau - T}$$

Once the new elimination rate constant (k) has been determined, the new volume of distribution (V_D) can be calculated to achieve the *desired* minimum and maximum concentrations as follows:

$$V_D = \frac{\frac{D}{T}(1 - e^{-kT})}{k(C_{max} - C_{min}e^{-kT})}$$

where D is the dose *previously given*, C_{max} and C_{min} are the *measured* serum concentrations, and T is the infusion time.

The adjusted values for volume of distribution and rate constant can be used to calculate the new dosing interval (τ) and dose (D) with the equations given in Steps 5 and 6.

Pharmacy Applications. Computer programs are available for calculating and monitoring a patient's aminoglycoside therapy, but the pharmacist should be able to calculate these parameters when the program is unavailable and also to ensure the accuracy of the dosing program.

EXAMPLE PROBLEMS

1. Gentamicin is chosen to treat a susceptible infection in a patient with the following characteristics:

Age: 63 years old

Weight: 142 lb

Height: 5′4″

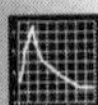

Gender: Female

Serum creatinine: 1.1 mg/dL

A. Calculate the gentamicin dosage regimen for this patient with a desired peak concentration of 6 μg/mL, a trough concentration of 1.5 μg/mL, and an infusion time of 1 hour.

$$\text{Weight} = 142 \text{ lb} \times \frac{1 \text{ kg}}{2.2 \text{ lb}} = 64.55 \text{ kg}$$

$$\text{IBW} = 45.5 \text{ kg} + 2.3 \text{ kg} \times 4 \text{ in} = 54.7 \text{ kg}$$

$$\text{IBW} \pm 30\% = 38.29 - 71.11 \text{ kg}$$

(The patient is within 30% of IBW.)

$$\text{CrCl} = 0.85 \times \frac{(140 - 63 \text{ yr}) \times 64.55 \text{ kg}}{72 \times 1.1 \text{ mg/dL}} = 53.34 \text{ mL/min}$$

$$k = 0.00293 \times 53.34 \text{ mL/min} + 0.014 = 0.17 \text{ hr}^{-1}$$

$$V_D = 0.26 \text{ L/kg} \times 64.55 \text{ kg} = 16.78 \text{ L}$$

$$\tau = \frac{\ln 6 \ \mu\text{g/mL} - \ln 1.5 \ \mu\text{g/mL}}{0.17 \text{ hr}^{-1}} + 1 \text{ hr} = 9.15 \text{ hr} \approx 8 \text{ hr}$$

$$D = 1 \text{ hr} \times (0.17 \text{ hr}^{-1}) \times (16.78 \text{ L}) \times (6 \text{ mg/L}) \times \left(\frac{1 - e^{-0.17 \text{ hr}^{-1}(8 \text{ hr})}}{1 - e^{-0.17 \text{ hr}^{-1}(1 \text{ hr})}}\right) = 81.38 \text{ mg} \approx 80 \text{ mg}$$

The patient should receive 80 mg of gentamicin every 8 hours.

B. How long until the patient reaches steady-state?

$$t_{1/2} = \frac{0.693}{0.17 \text{ hr}^{-1}} = 4.08 \text{ hr}$$

$$4.08 \text{ hr} \times 5 = 20.38 \text{ hr}$$

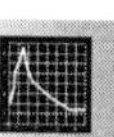

C. Approximately 24 hours after the first dose of gentamicin, blood samples are drawn from this patient and analyzed with a peak level of 4.8 μg/mL and a trough level of 0.9 μg/mL. Calculate a new dosage regimen for this patient.

$$k = \frac{\ln 4.8\ \mu g/mL - \ln 0.9\ \mu g/mL}{8\ hr - 1\ hr} = 0.24\ hr^{-1}$$

$$V_D = \frac{\frac{80\ mg}{1\ hr}(1 - e^{-0.24\ hr^{-1}(1\ hr)})}{0.24\ hr^{-1}\ [4.8\ mg/L - 0.9\ mg/L(e^{-0.24\ hr^{-1}(1\ hr)})]} = 17.38\ L$$

$$\tau = \frac{\ln 6\ \mu g/mL - \ln 1.5\ \mu g/mL}{0.24\ hr^{-1}} + 1\ hr$$

$$= 6.78\ hr \approx 6\ hr$$

$$D = 1\ hr \times (0.24\ hr^{-1}) \times (17.38\ L) \times (6\ mg/L) \times \left(\frac{1 - e^{-0.24\ hr^{-1}(6\ hr)}}{1 - e^{-0.24\ hr^{-1}(1\ hr)}}\right) = 89.5\ mg \approx 90\ mg$$

The patient's dosage regimen should be adjusted to 90 mg of gentamicin every 6 hours.

2. A 54-year-old male is to receive amikacin for a susceptible infection. He is 6′1″ tall and weighs 360 lb, and his measured creatinine clearance is 46.82 mL/min. Calculate the loading dose and dosage regimen for the patient to achieve a peak concentration of 25 μg/mL and a trough concentration of 5 μg/mL with an infusion time of 30 minutes.

$$\text{Weight} = 360\ lb \times \frac{1\ kg}{2.2\ lb} = 163.64\ kg$$

73″ (6′1″) − 60″ (5′) = 13″

IBW = 50 kg + 2.3 kg × 13 in = 79.9 kg

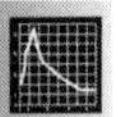

$$IBW \pm 30\% = 55.93 - 103.87 \text{ kg}$$

(The patient is NOT within 30% of IBW.)

$$k = 0.00293 \times 46.82 \text{ mL/min} + 0.014 = 0.151 \text{ hr}^{-1}$$

$$V_D = 0.26 \text{ L/kg} \times [79.9 \text{ kg} + 0.4(163.64 \text{ kg} - 79.9 \text{ kg})] = 29.48 \text{ L}$$

$$\tau = \frac{\ln 25 \ \mu\text{g/mL} - \ln 5 \ \mu\text{g/mL}}{0.151 \text{ hr}^{-1}} + 0.5 \text{ hr} = 11.16 \text{ hr} \approx 12 \text{ hr}$$

$$D = 0.5 \text{ hr} \times (0.151 \text{ hr}^{-1}) \times (29.48 \text{ L}) \times (25 \text{ mg/L}) \times \left(\frac{1 - e^{-0.151 \text{ hr}^{-1}(12 \text{ hr})}}{1 - e^{-0.151 \text{ hr}^{-1}(0.5 \text{ hr})}}\right) = 640.2 \text{ mg} \approx 640 \text{ mg}$$

$$LD = 25 \text{ mg/L} \times 29.48 \text{ L} = 737 \text{ mg} \approx 740 \text{ mg}$$

The patient should receive a 740-mg loading dose followed by 640 mg of amikacin every 12 hours.

17.2 Vancomycin

Vancomycin dosing, similar to aminoglycoside dosing presented in Section 17.1, must be individualized based on the patient's body weight, renal function, and measured serum concentrations of the drug.

Discussion. The pharmacokinetic parameters and dosage regimen for vancomycin can be calculated as follows[1]:

1. Calculate the patient's creatinine clearance (CrCl) using the Cockcroft-Gault equation and IBW.
2. Calculate the clearance (Cl, in mL/min/kg) based on the patient's weight (in kg) using the following equation:

$$Cl = 0.695 \times \frac{CrCl}{Weight} + 0.05$$

3. Determine the volume of distribution (V_D, in liters) as follows:

$$V_D = 0.7 \text{ L/kg} \times \text{Weight (in kg)}$$

4. Calculate the elimination rate constant (k, in hours^{-1}) using the following equation and the appropriate factors to convert to the necessary units:

$$k = \frac{Cl}{V_D}$$

5. The peak vancomycin concentration ($C_{max,ss}$) should fall within 20 to 40 μg/mL, and the trough concentration ($C_{min,ss}$) should fall within 5 to 15 μg/mL.[2] Choose appropriate target blood levels to treat the suspected pathogen but to avoid adverse reactions. The units of μg/mL are often used interchangeably with equivalent units of mg/L.
6. Calculate the dosing interval (τ, in hours) needed to achieve the concentrations chosen above using the following equation:

$$\tau = \frac{\ln C_{max,ss} - \ln C_{min,ss}}{k}$$

The value calculated for τ is usually rounded off to an acceptable dosing interval (e.g., 8, 12, 24 hours).

7. Calculate the dose (D, in mg) using the following formula:

$$D = V_D C_{max,ss} (1 - e^{-k\tau})$$

This dose is then rounded off to the nearest 50 to 100 mg.

8. If a loading dose (LD) is necessary, it can be calculated using the following equation:

$$LD = C_{max,ss} \times V_D$$

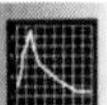

After this dosing regimen has been established for the patient, serum levels of vancomycin should be measured and the dose should be adjusted accordingly. To adjust the dose to achieve appropriate serum concentrations of the drug, whether or not the patient has reached steady-state should first be established. The patient is at steady-state after approximately three to five half-lives have passed, and the half-life ($t_{1/2}$) can be calculated using the following equation:

$$t_{1/2} = \frac{0.693}{k}$$

where k is the elimination rate constant calculated in Step 4 above.

If the patient has not reached steady-state, a serum vancomycin concentration should be obtained:

- Before a dose (C_{min})
- After an approximate 1-hour infusion of the drug followed by a 30-minute to 1-hour waiting time to allow for drug distribution (C_{max})
- Approximately one estimated half-life after C_{max} (C_3)

Using C_{max}, C_3, and the time elapsed between these measurements (Δt, in hours), the following calculation can be used to calculate a new elimination rate constant:

$$k = \frac{\ln C_{max} - \ln C_3}{\Delta t}$$

If the patient has reached steady-state, a serum vancomycin concentration should be obtained:

- Before a dose ($C_{min,ss}$)
- After an approximate 1-hour infusion of the drug followed by a 30-minute to 1-hour waiting time to allow for drug distribution ($C_{max,ss}$)

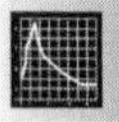

Using these two concentrations, the dosage interval (τ, in hours), and the infusion time plus waiting time (T_{max}, in hours), the following calculation can be used to calculate a new elimination rate constant:

$$k = \frac{\ln C_{max,ss} - \ln C_{min,ss}}{\tau - T_{max}}$$

Once the new elimination rate constant (k) has been determined, the new volume of distribution (V_D) can be calculated to achieve the *desired* minimum and maximum concentrations as follows:

$$V_D = \frac{D}{C_{max} - C_{min}}$$

where D is the dose *previously given* and C_{max} and C_{min} are the *measured* serum concentrations.

The adjusted values for volume of distribution and rate constant can be used to calculate the new dosing interval (τ) and dose (D) with the equations given in Steps 6 and 7.

EXAMPLE PROBLEMS

1. A 49-year-old female patient is admitted to the hospital with a methicillin-resistant *Staphylococcus aureus* infection. The patient is 5′7″ tall, weighs 63 kg, and has a serum creatinine of 0.85 mg/dL. Vancomycin infused over 1 hour is chosen to treat this infection, with target maximum and minimum serum concentrations established at 30 μg/mL and 10 μg/mL, respectively. Calculate the vancomycin half-life, loading dose, and appropriate dosage regimen for this patient.

IBW = 45.5 kg + 2.3 kg × 7 in = 61.6 kg

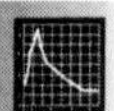

$$\text{IBW} \pm 30\% = 43.12 - 80.08 \text{ kg (The patient is within 30\% of IBW.)}$$

$$\text{CrCl} = 0.85 \times \frac{(140 - 49 \text{ yr}) \times 63 \text{ kg}}{72 \times 0.85 \text{ mg/dL}} = 79.63 \text{ mL/min}$$

$$\text{Cl} = 0.695 \times \frac{79.63 \text{ mL/min}}{63 \text{ kg}} + 0.05 = 0.928 \text{ mL/min/kg}$$

$$V_D = 0.7 \text{ L/kg} \times 63 \text{ kg} = 44.1 \text{ L}$$

$$k = \frac{\left(\frac{0.928 \text{ mL}}{1 \text{ min/kg}} \times \frac{1 \text{ L}}{1{,}000 \text{ mL}} \times \frac{60 \text{ min}}{1 \text{ hr}} \times 63 \text{ kg}\right)}{} = 0.0795 \text{ hr}^{-1}$$

$$t_{1/2} = \frac{0.693}{0.0795 \text{ hr}^{-1}} = 8.72 \text{ hr}$$

$$\tau = \frac{\ln 30 \ \mu\text{g/mL} - \ln 10 \ \mu\text{g/mL}}{0.0795 \text{ hr}^{-1}} = 13.82 \text{ hr} \approx 12 \text{ hr}$$

$$D = 44.1 \text{ L} \times 30 \text{ mg/L} \times (1 - e^{-0.0795 \text{ hr}^{-1}(12 \text{ hr})}) = 813.38 \text{ mg} \approx 800 \text{ mg}$$

$$LD = 30 \text{ mg/L} \times 44.1 \text{ L} = 1{,}323 \text{ mg} \approx 1{,}300 \text{ mg}$$

The patient should receive a 1,300-mg loading dose of vancomycin, followed by 800 mg every 12 hours.

2. Approximately 1 hour after the second dose, the patient in Example Problem 1 begins to experience some adverse reactions. A vancomycin level is checked 10 minutes before her third dose and analyzed at 18 μg/mL. Vancomycin levels are then checked at 30 minutes and 8 hours after the third infusion and analyzed at 46 μg/mL and 29 μg/mL, respectively. How should the patient's dosage regimen be adjusted to reach the determined peak and trough blood concentrations of 10 μg/mL and 30 μg/mL?

$8.72 \text{ hr} \times 3 = 26.16 \text{ hr}$

$8.72 \text{ hr} \times 5 = 43.6 \text{ hr}$

Although the blood levels were checked almost 36 hours after her first dose of vancomycin, it is not definite that the patient has reached steady-state because she has only received three doses of the drug. Therefore, it is best to use the equation for a patient not at steady-state.

$$k = \frac{\ln 46\ \mu\text{g/mL} - \ln 29\ \mu\text{g/mL}}{8\text{ hr} - 0.5\text{ hr}} = 0.0615\ \text{hr}^{-1}$$

$$V_D = \frac{800\text{ mg}}{46\text{ mg/L} - 18\text{ mg/L}} = 28.57\text{ L}$$

$$\tau = \frac{\ln 30\ \mu\text{g/mL} - \ln 10\ \mu\text{g/mL}}{0.0615\ \text{hr}^{-1}} = 17.86\text{ hr} \approx 18\text{ hr}$$

$$D = 28.57\text{ L} \times 30\text{ mg/L} \times (1 - e^{-0.0615\ \text{hr}^{-1}(18\ \text{hr})})$$
$$= 573.79\text{ mg} \approx 550\text{ mg}$$

The patient should receive 550 mg of vancomycin every 18 hours.

17.3 Digoxin

Digoxin doses are calculated by taking into account the patient's cardiac and renal function and disease state being treated. Furthermore, because digoxin is available in several different dosage forms, the bioavailability (F) must also be included for intravenous injection ($F = 1$), capsules ($F = 0.9$), tablets ($F = 0.7$), and elixir ($F = 0.8$).[1]

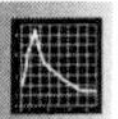

Discussion. The pharmacokinetic parameters and dosage regimen for digoxin can be calculated as follows[1]:

1. Calculate the patient's creatinine clearance (CrCl) using the Cockcroft-Gault equation.
2. Calculate digoxin clearance (Cl, in mL/min) using the following equation:

   $$Cl = 1.303 \times CrCl + Cl_m$$

   where Cl_m (metabolic clearance) = 40 mL/min in patients with no or mild heart failure or = 20 mL/min in patients with moderate to severe heart failure.
3. The volume of distribution (V_D, in liters) depends on renal function and is calculated as follows:

   $$V_D = 226 + \left(\frac{298 \times CrCl}{29.1 + CrCl}\right)$$

4. Choose an appropriate serum concentration (C_{ss}) value based on the disease state being treated. For the treatment of heart failure, the serum concentration is usually 1 ng/mL or less, and for the treatment of atrial fibrillation the serum concentration is usually 1 to 1.5 ng/mL.
5. The loading dose can be calculated using the volume of distribution and serum concentration as follows:

   $$LD = C_{ss} \times V_D$$

   The units for the loading dose are usually micrograms or milligrams; therefore, the appropriate conversion factors for C_{ss} are used to obtain the units desired. Half of the loading dose is usually given initially, followed by two more doses at one-fourth of the loading dose given at 4- to 6-hour intervals after assessing the patient's blood pressure, heart rate, and signs of adverse response to the digoxin.

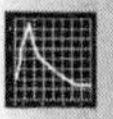

6. The dose (D) and dosing interval (τ) can then be calculated using the following equation:

$$\frac{D}{\tau} = \frac{C_{ss} \times Cl}{F}$$

As stated above, the units for the dose are usually micrograms or milligrams, and the dosing interval for the maintenance dose is usually 1 day. These units are achieved by using the appropriate conversion factors for C_{ss} and Cl. Also, the value for the dose may be rounded to an acceptable value.

In the case that a patient's steady-state blood concentration of digoxin is unacceptable ($C_{ss,old}$), the dose can be adjusted (D_{new}) to achieve the desired blood concentration ($C_{ss,new}$) using the following equation:

$$D_{new} = D_{old}\left(\frac{C_{ss,new}}{C_{ss,old}}\right)$$

EXAMPLE PROBLEMS

1. A 61-year-old female patient is experiencing mild heart failure. She is 5′0″ tall, weighs 128 lb, and has a serum creatinine concentration of 0.95 mg/dL.

A. Calculate the intravenous loading dose for achieving a serum digoxin concentration of 1 ng/mL. Also calculate the volume of digoxin injection with a concentration of 0.25 mg/mL needed for the loading dose.

$$\text{Weight} = 128 \text{ lb} \times \frac{1 \text{ kg}}{2.2 \text{ lb}} = 58.18 \text{ kg}$$

$$\text{CrCl} = 0.85 \times \frac{(140 - 61 \text{ yr}) \times 58.18 \text{ kg}}{72 \times 0.95 \text{ mg/dL}} = 57.12 \text{ mL/min}$$

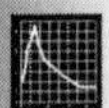

$$Cl = 1.303 \times 57.12 \text{ mL/min} + 40 \text{ mL/min} = 114.43 \text{ mL/min}$$

$$V_D = 226 + \left(\frac{298 \times 57.12 \text{ mL/min}}{29.1 + 57.12 \text{ mL/min}}\right) = 423.42 \text{ L}$$

$$LD = \frac{1 \text{ ng}}{1 \text{ mL}} \times \frac{1{,}000 \text{ mL}}{1 \text{ L}} \times \frac{1 \text{ µg}}{1{,}000 \text{ ng}} \times 423.42 \text{ L} = 423.42 \text{ µg} \approx 420 \text{ µg}$$

$$420 \text{ µg} \times 0.5 = 210 \text{ µg}$$

$$420 \text{ µg} \times 0.25 = 105 \text{ µg}$$

$$210 \text{ µg} \times \frac{1 \text{ mg}}{1{,}000 \text{ µg}} \times \frac{1 \text{ mL}}{0.25 \text{ mg}} = 0.84 \text{ mL}$$

$$105 \text{ µg} \times \frac{1 \text{ mg}}{1{,}000 \text{ µg}} \times \frac{1 \text{ mL}}{0.25 \text{ mg}} = 0.42 \text{ mL}$$

The patient should receive 0.84 mL of digoxin injection (210 µg digoxin) now, and 0.42 mL (105 µg) every 6 hours for two subsequent doses.

B. Calculate the maintenance dose to maintain the 1 ng/mL serum concentration and the number of tablets needed for this dose.

$$\frac{D}{\tau} = \frac{\left(\frac{1 \text{ ng}}{1 \text{ mL}} \times \frac{1 \text{ µg}}{1{,}000 \text{ ng}} \times \frac{114.43 \text{ mL}}{1 \text{ min}} \times \frac{60 \text{ min}}{1 \text{ hr}} \times \frac{24 \text{ hr}}{1 \text{ day}}\right)}{0.7}$$

$$= 235.4 \text{ µg/day}$$

The patient should receive one 250-µg (0.25-mg) tablet daily.

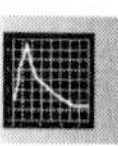

C. After taking one 0.25-mg tablet daily for 1 month, the patient begins to complain of adverse effects similar to those of digoxin toxicity. Her steady-state digoxin level was checked and reported by the laboratory as 1.8 ng/mL. How should her dose be adjusted to produce the desired blood level of 1 ng/mL?

$$D_{new} = 0.25 \text{ mg/day} \left(\frac{1 \text{ ng/mL}}{1.8 \text{ ng/mL}} \right) = 0.139 \text{ mg/day}$$

The patient should be switched to one 0.125-mg tablet daily and monitored to ensure that adequate blood levels are being attained at this dose.

2. Calculate the loading and maintenance doses for an 82-year-old male patient who is experiencing atrial fibrillation and severe heart failure. The patient weighs 141 lb, is 5′9″ tall, and has a serum creatinine concentration of 2.18 mg/dL. The desired digoxin serum concentration is 1.5 ng/mL, and capsules will be used to administer the maintenance doses.

$$\text{Weight} = 141 \text{ lb} \times \frac{1 \text{ kg}}{2.2 \text{ lb}} = 64.09 \text{ kg}$$

$$\text{CrCl} = \frac{(140 - 82 \text{ yr}) \times 64.09 \text{ kg}}{72 \times 2.18 \text{ mg/dL}} = 23.68 \text{ mL/min}$$

$$\text{Cl} = 1.303 \times 23.68 \text{ mL/min} + 20 \text{ mL/min} = 50.86 \text{ mL/min}$$

$$V_D = 226 + \left(\frac{298 \times 23.68 \text{ mL/min}}{29.1 + 23.68 \text{ mL/min}} \right) = 359.7 \text{ L}$$

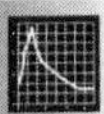

$$\text{LD} = \frac{1.5\text{ ng}}{1\text{ mL}} \times \frac{1{,}000\text{ mL}}{1\text{ L}} \times \frac{1\ \mu\text{g}}{1{,}000\text{ ng}} \times 359.7\text{ L}$$
$$= 539.55\ \mu\text{g} \approx 540\ \mu\text{g}$$

$540\ \mu g \times 0.5 = 270\ \mu g$

$540\ \mu g \times 0.25 = 135\ \mu g$

The patient should receive 270 μg of digoxin now, and 135 μg every 6 hours for two subsequent doses.

$$\frac{D}{\tau} = \frac{\left(\frac{1.5\text{ ng}}{1\text{ mL}} \times \frac{1\ \mu\text{g}}{1{,}000\text{ ng}} \times \frac{50.86\text{ mL}}{1\text{ min}} \times \frac{60\text{ min}}{1\text{ hr}} \times \frac{24\text{ hr}}{1\text{ day}}\right)}{0.9}$$

$$= 122.06\ \mu\text{g/day}$$

The patient should receive one 100-μg (0.1-mg) capsule daily.

17.4 Heparin

Heparin therapy must be closely monitored by evaluating the patient's activated partial thromboplastin time (aPTT) to avoid excessive bleeding. Heparin doses are adjusted frequently to produce the desired aPTT, which is approximately 46 to 70 seconds but varies by institution.

Discussion. The initial loading dose of heparin for treating or preventing deep vein thrombosis or pulmonary embolism is 80 units/kg (maximum of 10,000 units) followed by a continuous infusion of 18 units/kg/hr (maximum of 2,300 units/hr). To treat acute coronary syndromes, the heparin loading dose is 70 units/kg (maximum of 5,000 units) followed by a continuous infusion of 15 units/kg/hr (maximum of 1,000

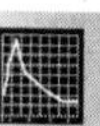

units/hr).[3,4] These doses are based on actual body weight in nonobese patients. For obese patients, the adjusted body weight should be used (see Section 13.1). Heparin reaches steady-state in approximately 6 hours; therefore, the evaluation of therapy by aPTT or other factors should occur at least 6 hours after initiation of or change in heparin therapy. Once the aPTT is measured, the heparin dose can be adjusted as follows[3,5]:

aPTT (sec)	Dose Adjustment
<35	80 units/kg bolus then increase infusion by 4 units/kg/hr
<35–45	40 units/kg bolus then increase infusion by 2 units/kg/hr
46–70	No change
71–90	Decrease infusion by 2 units/kg/hr
>90	Hold infusion for 1 hr then decrease by 3 units/kg/hr

The values given in this table may differ from the heparin protocol at a particular institution because of variations in clinical laboratory measurements of aPTT in that institution. If an institution has an established heparin protocol, it should be used instead of this table.

EXAMPLE PROBLEMS

1. A male patient weighing 76 kg and measuring 5′9″ tall is placed on heparin therapy for prevention of deep vein thrombosis after surgery.

A. How many milliliters of a heparin injectable solution containing 5,000 units/mL should be administered to this patient for a loading dose of 80 units/kg?

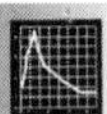

$$\text{IBW} = 50 \text{ kg} + 2.3 \text{ kg} \times 9 \text{ in} = 70.7 \text{ kg}$$

$$\text{IBW} \pm 30\% = 49.49 - 91.91 \text{ kg}$$

(The patient is within 30% of IBW.)

$$\frac{80 \text{ units}}{1 \text{ kg}} \times 76 \text{ kg} \times \frac{1 \text{ mL}}{5{,}000 \text{ units}} = 1.22 \text{ mL}$$

B. What would be the continuous infusion rate for this patient using a solution with a heparin concentration of 25,000 units/500 mL to administer 18 units/kg/hr?

$$\frac{18 \text{ units}}{1 \text{ kg/hr}} \times 76 \text{ kg} \times \frac{500 \text{ mL}}{25{,}000 \text{ units}}$$

$$= 27.36 \text{ mL/hr} \approx 27 \text{ mL/hr}$$

C. Six hours after the heparin therapy is initiated, a blood sample is drawn from this patient and the aPTT is found to be 88 seconds. How should the current infusion rate be adjusted to lower the patient's aPTT?

According to the table above, the infusion rate should be decreased by 2 units/kg/hr.

$$\frac{18 \text{ units}}{1 \text{ kg/hr}} - \frac{2 \text{ units}}{1 \text{ kg/hr}} = \frac{16 \text{ units}}{1 \text{ kg/hr}}$$

$$\frac{16 \text{ units}}{1 \text{ kg/hr}} \times 76 \text{ kg} \times \frac{500 \text{ mL}}{25{,}000 \text{ units}}$$

$$= 24.32 \text{ mL/hr} \approx 24 \text{ mL/hr}$$

The current infusion rate of 27 mL/hr should be decreased to 24 mL/hr.

2. A female patient with acute coronary syndrome is to begin heparin therapy. This 144-lb, 5′1″ tall patient should receive a bolus dose of 70 units/kg followed by an infusion of 15 units/kg/hr.

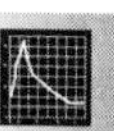

A. How many milliliters of a heparin injectable solution containing 2,000 units/mL should be administered to this patient for the loading dose, and what would be the continuous infusion rate for this patient using a solution with a heparin concentration of 10,000 units/500 mL?

$$144 \text{ lb} \times \frac{1 \text{ kg}}{2.2 \text{ lb}} = 65.45 \text{ kg}$$

$$\text{IBW} = 45.5 \text{ kg} + 2.3 \text{ kg} \times 1 \text{ in} = 47.8 \text{ kg}$$

$$\text{IBW} + 30\% = 62.14 \text{ kg}$$

(Patient's weight is greater than 30% of IBW.)

Adjusted body weight =

$$[(65.45 \text{ kg} - 47.8 \text{ kg}) \times 0.2] + 47.8 \text{ kg} = 51.33 \text{ kg}$$

$$\frac{70 \text{ units}}{1 \text{ kg}} \times 51.33 \text{ kg} \times \frac{1 \text{ mL}}{2{,}000 \text{ units}} = 1.8 \text{ mL}$$

$$\frac{15 \text{ units}}{1 \text{ kg/hr}} \times 51.33 \text{ kg} \times \frac{500 \text{ mL}}{10{,}000 \text{ units}} = 38.498 \text{ mL/hr} \approx 38 \text{ mL/hr}$$

The patient should receive a loading dose of 1.8 mL and a continuous infusion of heparin at a rate of 38 mL/hr.

B. A blood sample taken from the patient approximately 6 hours after the heparin therapy is initiated shows an aPTT of 24 seconds. How should the current heparin therapy be adjusted to bring the patient's aPTT to within normal limits?

According to the table, the patient should receive a bolus dose of 80 units/kg and the infusion rate should be increased by 4 units/kg/hr.

$$\frac{80 \text{ units}}{1 \text{ kg}} \times 51.33 \text{ kg} \times \frac{1 \text{ mL}}{2{,}000 \text{ units}} = 2.05 \text{ mL}$$

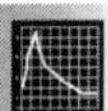

$$\frac{15 \text{ units}}{1 \text{ kg/hr}} + \frac{4 \text{ units}}{1 \text{ kg/hr}} = \frac{19 \text{ units}}{1 \text{ kg/hr}}$$

$$\frac{19 \text{ units}}{1 \text{ kg/hr}} \times 51.33 \text{ kg} \times \frac{500 \text{ mL}}{10{,}000 \text{ units}} = 48.76 \text{ mL/hr} \approx 49 \text{ mL/hr}$$

The patient should receive a bolus dose of 2.05 mL of the 2,000 units/mL solution, and the current infusion rate of 38 mL/hr should be increased to 49 mL/hr.

17.5 Warfarin

Warfarin therapy is monitored based on a patient's prothrombin time (PT) to ensure adequate anticoagulation therapy without potential for excessive bleeding. Thromboplastin variations may cause discrepancies in a patient's PT analyzed in the laboratory. Therefore, an International Sensitivity Index (ISI), which is a measure of the thromboplastin's responsiveness compared with the World Health Organization reference standard, is used to convert the PT to the International Normalized Ratio (INR) by the following equation[6]:

$$\text{INR} = \left(\frac{\text{PT}_{\text{patient}}}{\text{PT}_{\text{control}}}\right)^{\text{ISI}}$$

This calculation is usually performed in the laboratory where the PT is analyzed. The goal INR value for the prevention or treatment of most thromboembolic disease is 2.5 with a range of 2.0 to 3.0.

Discussion. Most patients can be initiated at a warfarin dose of 4 to 5 mg/day, unless the patient is sensitive to warfarin, for example, elderly patients more than 75 years old or patients receiving drugs that interact with warfarin. Evaluation of the patient's warfarin therapy

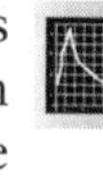

by monitoring INR should be performed as often as daily while dosage adjustments are being made and can be extended to every 4 to 6 weeks after the appropriate dosage regimen has been established. To adjust warfarin therapy to deliver an appropriate dose for a patient, the following table may be used[6]:

INR	Dose Adjustment
<2.0	Increase by 5%–15%
2.0–3.0	No change
3.1–3.5	Decrease by 5%–15%
3.6–4.0	May hold one dose, decrease by 10%–15%
>4.0	May hold one to two doses, decrease by 10%–15%

EXAMPLE PROBLEMS

1. A patient is started on a dose of 4 mg of warfarin daily, and approximately 24 hours after the initial dose, the patient's INR is 0.8.

A. What is the next dose of warfarin that should be given?

According to the table, the dose should be increased by 5% to 15%.

$4 \text{ mg/day} \times 5\% = 0.2 \text{ mg/day}$

$4 \text{ mg/day} \times 15\% = 0.6 \text{ mg/day}$

The patient should receive 4.2 to 4.6 mg/day. To achieve a dose of 4.5 mg/day, the patient should take one 2-mg tablet and one 2.5-mg tablet.

B. Approximately 24 hours after receiving the 4.5-mg dose, the patient's INR is 1.5. What dose of warfarin should be given?

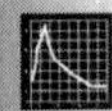

4.5 mg/day × 5% = 0.23 mg

4.5 mg/day × 15% = 0.68 mg

The patient should receive 4.73 to 5.18 mg/day, and thus should take one 5-mg tablet.

2. A patient has been taking one 7.5-mg warfarin tablet daily for several months and comes in for his annual physical exam. His blood sample reveals an INR of 3.7. How should his warfarin dose be adjusted?

   According to the table, the dose should be decreased by 10% to 15%, and the patient may need to skip the next dose.

   7.5 mg/day × 10% = 0.75 mg

   7.5 mg/day × 15% = 1.13 mg

   The patient's dose should be decreased to 6.37–6.75 mg daily. Because the next lower tablet strength is 6 mg, the patient may take a 6-mg tablet for his next dose and then alternate with a 7.5-mg tablet every other day to receive an average dose of 6.75 mg/day.

17.6 Iron

Iron preparations are used to treat iron-deficient anemia, and in most patients, approximately 200 mg of elemental iron daily given orally in divided doses will successfully treat the anemia.[7] However, oral iron products cannot be used in cases of iron malabsorption or intolerance, and a parenteral product must be used. Iron is administered intramuscularly or intravenously in the form of iron dextran and is available as a solution that provides 50 mg of elemental iron per milliliter.

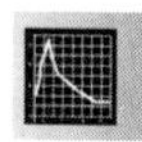

Discussion. There are two methods for calculating the amount of iron dextran to administer to a patient based on his or her measured hemoglobin level (Hgb). The first method produces the volume of iron dextran solution to administer using the following equation[2]:

$$\text{Dose (mL)} = 0.0442\,(\text{desired Hgb} - \text{observed Hgb}) \times \text{IBW} + (0.26 \times \text{IBW})$$

This equation can be used for adults and children weighing more than 15 kg (33 lb); however, if the actual body weight is less than the IBW, the actual weight should be used. This equation can also be applied to children weighing 5 to 15 kg (11 to 33 lb), with the actual weight in kilograms used. The desired Hgb range for female patients is 12.1–15.3 g/dL and for male patients is 13.8–17.5 g/dL.[2]

The second method produces the amount of iron to be administered in the form of iron dextran based on the patient's body weight in pounds and an average Hgb of 14.8 g/dL using the following equation[8]:

$$\text{Iron (mg)} = \text{Weight (lb)} \times 0.3 \times \left(100 - \frac{\text{Hgb} \times 100}{14.8}\right)$$

The result of this equation then must be converted to the volume of iron dextran solution to administer by dividing the amount of iron by 50 mg/mL.

In patients who are anemic because of blood loss, the following equation based on the volume of blood lost (in milliliters) and the patient's hematocrit (expressed as a decimal fraction) may be used[8]:

$$\text{Iron (mg)} = \text{Blood loss} \times \text{Hematocrit}$$

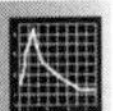

As stated above, the volume of iron dextran solution to administer is determined by dividing the amount of iron by 50 mg/mL.

EXAMPLE PROBLEMS

1. A 22-year-old female patient weighing 110 pounds and measuring 5′3″ has an Hgb of 9.2 g/dL. Using the first method described above, calculate the amount of iron dextran solution to administer to this patient to reach an Hgb concentration of 15 g/dL.

$$\text{IBW} = 45.5 \text{ kg} + 2.3 \text{ kg} \times 3 \text{ in} = 52.4 \text{ kg}$$

$$\text{Weight} = 110 \text{ lb} \times \frac{1 \text{ kg}}{2.2 \text{ lb}} = 50 \text{ kg}$$

Because the patient's actual body weight is less than her IBW, her actual body weight should be used.

$$\text{Dose} = 0.0442\,(15 \text{ g/dL} - 9.2 \text{ g/dL}) \times 50 \text{ kg} + (0.26 \times 50 \text{ kg}) = 25.82 \text{ mL}$$

2. An 85-year-old male patient weighing 176 lb has a measured Hgb level of 7.6 g/dL. Using the second method described above, calculate the volume of iron dextran solution to administer to this patient.

$$\text{Iron} = 176 \text{ lb} \times 0.3 \times \left(100 - \frac{7.6 \text{ g/dL} \times 100}{14.8}\right) = 2{,}568.65 \text{ mg}$$

$$\text{Volume} = 2{,}568.65 \text{ mg} \times \frac{1 \text{ mL}}{50 \text{ mg}} = 51.37 \text{ mL}$$

3. A patient is estimated to have lost 2 pints of blood due to a duodenal ulcer, and his measured hematocrit is 25.6%. What volume of iron dextran solution should be administered to replace the iron in the blood lost?

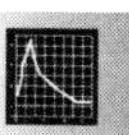

$$\text{Iron} = 2 \text{ pints} \times \frac{473 \text{ mL}}{1 \text{ pint}} \times 0.256 = 242.18 \text{ mg}$$

$$\text{Volume} = 242.18 \text{ mg} \times \frac{1 \text{ mL}}{50 \text{ mg}} = 4.84 \text{ mL}$$

17.7 Theophylline

Theophylline dosing is dependent on the age of the patient, whether or not the patient uses tobacco products, and the patient's cardiac and hepatic function.

Discussion. Theophylline serum concentrations of 10 to 20 μg/mL are considered to be optimal.[2] Intravenous administration of theophylline can be calculated using an average volume of distribution of 0.5 L/kg as follows:[1]

1. Calculate the intravenous loading dose (LD) of theophylline using the patient's volume of distribution (V_D, 0.5 L/kg × Weight) and desired serum concentration (C_{ss}) as follows:

   $$LD = C_{ss} \times V_D$$

2. Calculate the clearance (Cl, in mL/hr or L/hr) by using the following table based on the patient's age, clinical condition, and weight:[9]

Age/Condition	Mean Clearance (mL/min/kg)
Children 1–9 years old	1.44
Children 9–12 years old or adult smokers	1.26
Children 12–16 years old or elderly smokers (>65 years old)	0.9
Adult nonsmokers	0.72
Elderly nonsmokers (>65 years old)	0.54
Decompensated CHF, cor pulmonale, cirrhosis	0.36

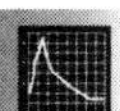

3. Determine the continuous infusion rate (k_0, in mg/hr) based on the desired serum concentration and clearance using the following equation:

$$k_0 = C_{ss} \times Cl$$

For oral doses of theophylline, the following chart based on the patient's age and clinical condition may be used[2]:

Age/Condition	Oral Loading Dose	Oral Maintenance Dose
Children 1–9 years old	5 mg/kg	4 mg/kg q6h
Children 9–16 years old or adult smokers	5 mg/kg	3 mg/kg q6h
Adult nonsmokers	5 mg/kg	3 mg/kg q8h
Elderly nonsmokers (>65 years old), patients with cor pulmonale	5 mg/kg	2 mg/kg q8h
Patients with CHF	5 mg/kg	1–2 mg/kg q12h

For any dosage form of theophylline, the dose can be adjusted to achieve a desired blood concentration ($C_{ss,new}$) if the measured blood concentration at steady-state ($C_{ss,old}$) is unacceptable. The new dose (D_{new}) can be calculated using the previous dose (D_{old}) and the blood levels as follows:

$$D_{new} = D_{old}\left(\frac{C_{ss,new}}{C_{ss,old}}\right)$$

If aminophylline (theophylline ethylenediamine) is to be used, the dose should be divided by 0.79 to account for the fact that approximately 79% of a dose of aminophylline is converted to theophylline.[10]

EXAMPLE PROBLEMS

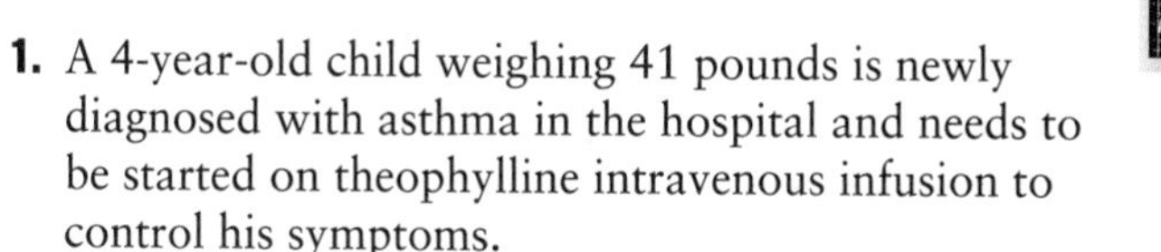

1. A 4-year-old child weighing 41 pounds is newly diagnosed with asthma in the hospital and needs to be started on theophylline intravenous infusion to control his symptoms.

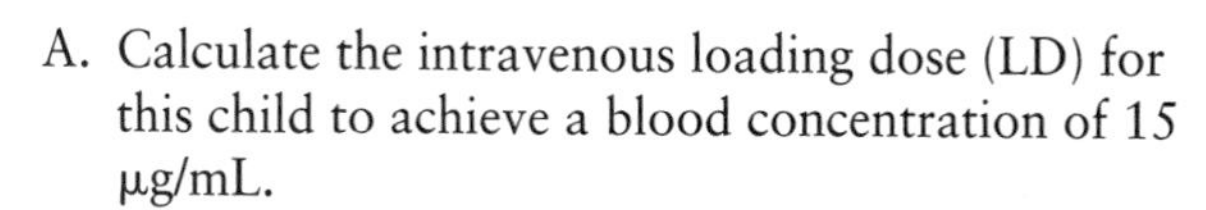

   A. Calculate the intravenous loading dose (LD) for this child to achieve a blood concentration of 15 μg/mL.

$$\text{Weight} = 41 \text{ lb} \times \frac{1 \text{ kg}}{2.2 \text{ lb}} = 18.64 \text{ kg}$$

$$V_D = \frac{0.5 \text{ L}}{1 \text{ kg}} \times 18.64 \text{ kg} = 9.32 \text{ L}$$

$$LD = \frac{15\ \mu\text{g}}{1 \text{ mL}} \times \frac{1{,}000 \text{ mL}}{1 \text{ L}} \times \frac{1 \text{ mg}}{1{,}000\ \mu\text{g}} \times 9.32 \text{ L} = 139.8 \text{ mg}$$

   B. Calculate the infusion rate in mL/hr for this child using an intravenous solution with a theophylline concentration of 2 mg/mL.

   Using the table in Step 2, the mean clearance for a 4-year-old child would be 1.44 mL/min/kg. Therefore, the clearance for this patient would be:

$$Cl = \frac{1.44 \text{ mL}}{1 \text{ min/kg}} \times 18.64 \text{ kg} \times \frac{60 \text{ min}}{1 \text{ hr}} = 1{,}610.18 \text{ mL/hr}$$

$$k_0 = \frac{15\ \mu\text{g}}{1 \text{ mL}} \times \frac{1 \text{ mg}}{1{,}000\ \mu\text{g}} \times \frac{1{,}610.18 \text{ mL}}{1 \text{ hr}} = 24.15 \text{ mg/hr}$$

$$\frac{24.15 \text{ mg}}{1 \text{ hr}} \times \frac{1 \text{ mL}}{2 \text{ mg}} = 12.08 \text{ mL/hr} \approx 12 \text{ mL/hr}$$

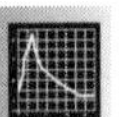

2. A 68-year-old nonsmoking female patient weighing 156 lb is to be started on aminophylline therapy.

A. Calculate the loading dose (LD) and continuous infusion rate of aminophylline to produce a theophylline serum concentration of 12 μg/mL.

$$\text{Weight} = 156 \text{ lb} \times \frac{1 \text{ kg}}{2.2 \text{ lb}} = 70.91 \text{ kg}$$

$$V_D = \frac{0.5 \text{ L}}{1 \text{ kg}} \times 70.91 \text{ kg} = 35.46 \text{ L}$$

$$LD = \frac{12\ \mu\text{g}}{1 \text{ mL}} \times \frac{1{,}000 \text{ mL}}{1 \text{ L}} \times \frac{1 \text{ mg}}{1{,}000\ \mu\text{g}} \times 35.46 \text{ L} = 425.52 \text{ mg}$$

$$\frac{425.52 \text{ mg theophylline}}{0.79} = 538.63 \text{ mg aminophylline}$$

$$Cl = \frac{0.54 \text{ mL}}{1 \text{ min/kg}} \times 70.91 \text{ kg} \times \frac{60 \text{ min}}{1 \text{ hr}} = 2{,}297.45 \text{ mL/hr}$$

$$k_0 = \frac{12\ \mu\text{g}}{1 \text{ mL}} \times \frac{1 \text{ mg}}{1{,}000\ \mu\text{g}} \times \frac{2{,}297.45 \text{ mL}}{1 \text{ hr}} = 27.57 \text{ mg/hr}$$

$$\frac{27.57 \text{ mg/hr}}{0.79} = 34.9 \text{ mg/hr}$$

B. The patient is to be sent home from the hospital on oral theophylline. Calculate an oral theophylline dosage regimen for this patient.

This patient should receive a dose of 2 mg/kg every 8 hours according to the table in the discussion section. Therefore, the dose for this patient would be:

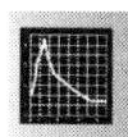

$$\frac{2\ \text{mg}}{1\ \text{kg}} \times 70.91\ \text{kg} = 141.82\ \text{mg q8h}$$

To achieve this dose, the patient could take one-half of a 300-mg tablet (not sustained-release) every 8 hours.

C. After 6 months of therapy, blood levels are drawn for this patient and analyzed for theophylline content. The results produce a theophylline concentration of 8 μg/mL. How should this patient's dose be adjusted to produce the desired serum concentration of 12 μg/mL?

$$D_{new} = 150\ \text{mg}\left(\frac{12\ \mu\text{g/mL}}{8\ \mu\text{g/mL}}\right) = 225\ \text{mg}$$

The patient's dose should be changed to one 200-mg tablet every 8 hours.

References

1. Dipiro JT, Talbert RL, Yee GC, Matzke GR, Wells BG, Posey LM, eds. Pharmacotherapy: A Pathophysiologic Approach, 5th Ed. New York, NY: McGraw-Hill, 2002: 41–49.
2. CliniSphere 2.0 [book on CD rom]. St. Louis, MO: Facts and Comparisons, 2002.
3. Hirsh J, Warkentin TE, Shaughnessy SG, et al. Heparin and low-molecular-weight heparin: mechanisms of action, pharmacokinetics, dosing, monitoring, efficacy, and safety. Chest 2002;119:64S–94S.
4. Dipiro JT, Talbert RL, Yee GC, Matzke GR, Wells BG, Posey LM, eds. Pharmacotherapy: A Pathophysiologic Approach, 5th Ed. New York, NY: McGraw-Hill, 2002:346.
5. Raschke RA, Reilly BM, Guidry JR, Fontana JR, Srinivas S. The weight-based heparin dosing nomogram compared with a "standard care" nomogram. Annals of Internal Medicine 1993;119:874–881.

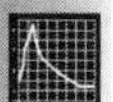

6. Koda-Kimble MA, Young LY, eds. Applied Therapeutics: The Clinical Use of Drugs, 7th ed. Baltimore, MD: Lippincott Williams & Wilkins, 2001:14.6–14.21.
7. Dipiro JT, Talbert RL, Yee GC, Matzke GR, Wells BG, Posey LM, eds. Pharmacotherapy: A Pathophysiologic Approach, 5th Ed. New York, NY: McGraw-Hill, 2002: 1736.
8. Koda-Kimble MA, Young LY, eds. Applied Therapeutics: The Clinical Use of Drugs. 7th ed. Baltimore, MD: Lippincott Williams & Wilkins, 2001:84.8.
9. Evans WE, Schentag JJ, Jusko WJ, eds. Applied Pharmacokinetics: Principles of Therapeutic Drug Monitoring. Vancouver, WA: Applied Therapeutics, 1992:13–22.
10. Genarro AR, ed. Remington: The Science & Practice of Pharmacy, 20th Ed. Baltimore, MD: Lippincott Williams & Wilkins, 2000:1298.

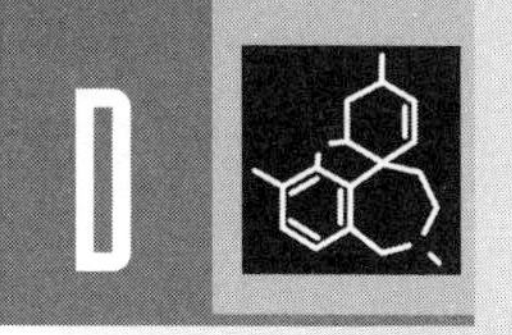

Chemical and Physical Calculations

18 SOME CHEMICAL CALCULATIONS

Situations may arise in some areas of pharmacy practice in which the pharmacist must perform calculations based on chemical properties of a drug. The topics discussed in this chapter, chemical stability and active drug moiety, are commonly seen especially in the area of compounding.

18.1 Chemical Stability

All drugs undergo chemical degradation over time, and the rate at which this degradation occurs is important in determining the length of time that the drug maintains its potency.

Definition. The chemical stability of a drug is the length of time that it retains its chemical integrity and labeled potency within the limits specified by the *United States Pharmacopeia* (USP).[1]

Expression. The stability of a drug is usually expressed as a length of time, which can then be used to establish an expiration date or "beyond-use" date.

Discussion. The chemical stability of a drug can be determined using chemical kinetics, and when considering

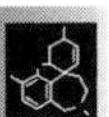

the stability of a drug, the reaction order and reaction rate must be investigated. Most drugs and excipients degrade by zero-order and first-order reactions,[1] and will therefore be the only reaction orders covered in this section. In equations pertaining to chemical kinetics, four variables are often encountered:

t—the amount of time that has passed
k—the reaction rate constant
C_t—drug concentration at time t
C_0—initial drug concentration

The units for C_t and C_0 are concentration units (e.g., mg/mL) or occasionally weight units (e.g., mg), and the units for k depend on the reaction order, as discussed in the following paragraphs. In determining the reaction order, a graph of drug concentration versus time must be constructed. If a straight line is formed by this graph, the reaction is zero-order. If a straight line is not formed, a graph of the natural logarithm (ln) of the drug concentration versus time should be constructed. If a straight line is formed by this graph, it confirms that the reaction follows first-order kinetics. In either case, the reaction rate constant (k) is the negative slope of the line formed by the graph of concentration versus time or natural log concentration versus time.

In zero-order reactions, the reaction rate is independent of concentration and remains constant over time. The equation used for zero-order reactions is:

$$C_t = -kt + C_0$$

The units for k are concentration per unit time (e.g., mg/mL/hr) or amount per unit time (e.g., mg/hr). In general, the reaction rate constant expresses the amount of drug that is lost per unit time.

In first-order reactions, the reaction rate is directly proportional to the remaining concentration with regard to time. The equation used for first-order reactions is:

$$\ln C_t = -kt + \ln C_0$$

The units for k are reciprocal time (e.g., hr^{-1}), and unlike zero-order reactions, k does not directly express the amount of drug lost per unit time.

Regardless of whether the reaction follows zero-order or first-order, the reaction rate constant is dependent on temperature. The following equation can be used to calculate the reaction rate constant (k_2) at a certain temperature (T_2) when the reaction rate constant (k_1) at a given temperature (T_1) is known:

$$\log \frac{k_2}{k_1} = \frac{E_a}{2.303\ R}\left(\frac{1}{T_1} - \frac{1}{T_2}\right)$$

where E_a is the activation energy for the reaction and R is the gas constant (1.987 cal/K mol or 8.314 J/K mol).

The temperatures in this equation are expressed in degrees Kelvin, which are calculated by adding 273 to the temperature in degrees Celsius. This equation is often used to shorten the duration of drug stability studies by allowing the drug to degrade quickly and determining k_1 at an elevated temperature, then calculating k_2 at room temperature.

Another, and perhaps more practical, equation for estimating changes in reaction rates based on temperature is as follows:[1]

$$t_{90,T2} = \frac{t_{90,T1}}{Q_{10}^{\frac{\Delta T}{10}}}$$

In this equation, Q_{10} is based on the activation energy of the reaction and can be calculated as a ratio of two reac-

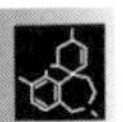

tion rate constants. However, because the activation energy and reaction rate constants may not be readily available to the pharmacist, Q_{10} values of 2, 3, or 4 corresponding to activation energies of 12.2, 19.4, or 24.5 kcal/mol can be used, and practical estimates can frequently be made using a value of 3. The known stability of the drug is $t_{90,T1}$; for example, cephalexin suspension is stable for approximately 14 days in the refrigerator. Furthermore, ΔT is $T_2 - T_1$ where T_1 is the temperature in degrees Celsius at which the stability is known and T_2 is the temperature in degrees Celsius for the unknown stability. This method, known as the Q_{10} method, can be used to *estimate* the effect of temperature on shelf-life and should not be substituted for complete stability studies.

Key Point. Chemical stability of a drug determines its shelf life and expiration date at a given temperature, which will change with variations in temperature.

Pharmacy Applications. Many times a pharmacist will be faced with questions regarding alternate storage conditions. The pharmacist can use his or her knowledge of chemical stability to make educated decisions regarding whether or not the drug can still be used by the patient. In addition, when a pharmacist uses one dosage form to compound another, the stability of the drug may change. The pharmacist may then need to perform a stability study to establish the correct shelf-life of the compounded preparation.

EXAMPLE PROBLEMS

1. A batch of transdermal patches containing 0.04 mg of drug each are prepared and stored at 25°C to test the stability at room temperature. Sample patches are analyzed periodically for the amount of drug

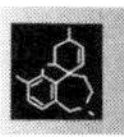

remaining, and the data represents a zero-order reaction with a rate constant of 0.0016 mg/month.

A. If this drug is said to maintain its potency until 92.5% of its original concentration is remaining, what would be the expiration date on patches that are manufactured on July 6?

$$C_t = 0.04 \text{ mg} \times 0.925 = 0.037 \text{ mg}$$

$$0.037 \text{ mg} = -0.0016 \text{ mg/mo} \times t + 0.04 \text{ mg}$$

$$t = 1.875 \text{ mo} \approx 1 \text{ mo } 26.25 \text{ days}$$

The patches will expire on September 1.

B. How much drug would be remaining after storage for 1 year and 2 months?

$$1 \text{ yr } 2 \text{ mo} = 14 \text{ mo}$$

$$C_t = -0.0016 \text{ mg/mo} \times 14 \text{ mo} + 0.04 \text{ mg} = 0.0176 \text{ mg}$$

2. A drug solution for intravenous administration containing 800 mg of drug per liter is prepared and stored at 25°C to test its stability. Samples are drawn periodically and analyzed using HPLC to determine the concentration. When graphed as a natural logarithm of concentration versus time, the data form a straight line with a slope of −0.09 week^{-1}. What will be the predicted concentration of the drug after 2 years at 25°C?

$$t = 2 \text{ yr} \times \frac{52 \text{ wk}}{1 \text{ yr}} = 104 \text{ wk}$$

$$\ln C_t = -0.09 \text{ week}^{-1} \times 104 \text{ wk} + \ln 800 \text{ mg/L} = -2.675$$

$$C_t = 0.069 \text{ mg/L}$$

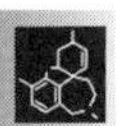

3. An accelerated stability study is performed at 75°C for a new drug. The first-order reaction rate constant at this temperature is found to be 0.15 yr^{-1}. The activation energy is 14.81 kJ/mol.

A. What would be the reaction rate constant at room temperature (approximately 25°C)?

$$k_1 = 0.15\ yr^{-1}$$

$$T_1 = 75°C + 273 = 348\ K$$

$$E_a = 14.81\ kJ/mol = 14{,}810\ J/mol$$

$$T_2 = 25°C + 273 = 298\ K$$

$$\log \frac{k_2}{0.15\ yr^{-1}} = \frac{14{,}810\ J/mol}{2.303 \times 8.314\ J/mol\ K} \times \left(\frac{1}{348\ K} - \frac{1}{298\ K}\right) = -0.373$$

$$\frac{k_2}{0.15\ yr^{-1}} = 0.424$$

$$k_2 = 0.064\ yr^{-1}$$

B. If the initial concentration of the drug is 2 mg/mL, how long would it take for the drug to reach 95% of its initial concentration at both 25°C and 75°C?

$$2\ mg/mL \times 95\% = 1.9\ mg/mL$$

At 75°C:

$$\ln 1.9\ mg/mL = -0.15\ yr^{-1} \times t + \ln 2\ mg/mL$$

$$t = 0.34\ yr = 4.1\ mo$$

At 25°C:

$$\ln 1.9\ mg/mL = -0.064\ yr^{-1} \times t + \ln 2\ mg/mL$$

$$t = 0.81\ yr = 9.68\ mo$$

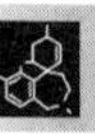

4. A pharmacist goes to work on a Monday morning in August and finds that the refrigerator is off. After some investigation, she finds that the electricity went off at 7:00 Friday evening and was just restored that morning before she came in (so the air conditioning was off as well). It was approximately 98°F on Saturday and Sunday. Ignoring fluctuations in temperature at night, estimate the stability of a drug that is stable for 28 days in the refrigerator at 5°C.

$$T_1 = 5°C$$

$$T_2 = 98°F = \frac{5}{9} \times (98° - 32°) = 36.67°C$$

$$\Delta T = 36.67°C - 5°C = 31.67°C$$

$$t_{90,T1} = 28 \text{ days}$$

$$t_{90,T2} = \frac{28 \text{ days}}{3^{\frac{31.67}{10}}} = 0.86 \text{ day} \times \frac{24 \text{ hr}}{1 \text{ day}}$$

$$= 20.72 \text{ hr}$$

5. An extemporaneously compounded suspension of a drug is stable for 6 months at room temperature (approximately 25°C). How long will it be stable in the refrigerator (approximately 5°C)?

$$T_1 = 25°C$$

$$T_2 = 5°C$$

$$\Delta T = 5°C - 25°C = -20°C$$

$$t_{90,T2} = \frac{6 \text{ mo}}{3^{\frac{-20}{10}}} = 54 \text{ mo} \times \frac{1 \text{ yr}}{12 \text{ mo}} = 4.5 \text{ yr}$$

18.2 Active Drug Moiety

It is sometimes necessary to calculate the amount of a pharmacologically active drug moiety when present as a salt, ester, hydrate, or complex chemical form.

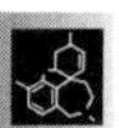

Definition. The *active drug moiety* is that portion of a chemical compound that is responsible for the compound's primary pharmacologic activity.

Discussion. The USP describes occasions in which a dose of a drug is specified in terms of a cation (e.g., Li^+), an anion (e.g., F^-), or a molecule (e.g., theophylline in theophylline ethylenediamine), and the exact amount of the salt or chemical complex to use must be calculated.[2] The calculations required involve application of atomic and molecular weights. For reference, a list of atomic weights is included in Appendix D.

To calculate the weight of a constituent in a given weight of a compound, the constituent's formula weight is related to the molecular weight of the compound. For example, to calculate the milligrams of lithium in 300 mg of lithium carbonate, the formula weight of lithium is compared to the molecular weight of lithium carbonate:

$$\text{Formula weight, Li} = 7 \text{ (atomic weight)} \times 2 \text{ (number of Li ions/molecule)} = 14$$

$$\text{Molecular weight, } Li_2CO_3 = 74$$

$$\frac{14 \text{ g/mole Li}}{74 \text{ g/mole } Li_2CO_3} \times 300 \text{ mg } Li_2CO_3 = 56.7 \text{ mg Li}$$

As another example, to calculate the number of milligrams of methadone (molecular weight, 313) in a solution containing 10 mg of methadone hydrochloride (molecular weight, 349):

$$\frac{313 \text{ g/mole methadone}}{349 \text{ g/mole methadone HCl}} \times 10 \text{ mg methadone HCl} = 8.97 \text{ mg methadone}$$

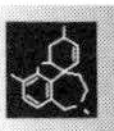

EXAMPLE PROBLEMS

1. A prescription calls for the preparation of 30 mL of a 1% solution of lidocaine (molecular weight, 234). For purposes of solubility, a pharmacist uses lidocaine hydrochloride (molecular weight, 288). How many milligrams of the latter should be used?

$$\frac{1\text{ g}}{100\text{ mL}} \times \frac{1{,}000\text{ mg}}{1\text{ g}} \times 30\text{ mL lidocaine} \times \frac{288\text{ g/mole lidocaine HCl}}{234\text{ g/mole lidocaine}} = 369.23\text{ mg lidocaine HCl}$$

2. How many milligrams of sodium fluoride (NaF) will provide 500 μg of fluoride ion?

Atomic weights: Na 23; F 19

$$\frac{42\text{ g/mole NaF}}{19\text{ g/mole F}} \times \frac{1\text{ mg}}{1{,}000\ \mu\text{g}} \times 500\ \mu\text{g F} = 1.11\text{ mg NaF}$$

3. How many milligrams of betamethasone diproprionate (molecular weight, 504) should be used to prepare a 50-g tube of ointment prescribed to contain the equivalent of 0.5 mg of betamethasone (molecular weight, 392) base per gram?

$$\frac{0.5\text{ mg betamethasone}}{1\text{ g}} \times \frac{504\text{ g/mole betamethasone diproprionate}}{392\text{ g/mole betamethasone}} \times 50\text{ g} = 32.14\text{ mg betamethasone diproprionate}$$

4. A sterile ophthalmic suspension of Betoptic S contains the equivalent of 0.25% of betaxolol

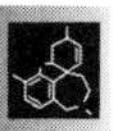

(molecular weight, 307), present as the hydrochloride salt (molecular weight, 344). Calculate the percent strength of betaxolol hydrochloride in the suspension.

$$\frac{0.25 \text{ g betaxolol}}{100 \text{ mL}} \times \frac{344 \text{ g/mole betaxolol HCl}}{307 \text{ g/mole betaxolol}}$$
$$= 0.28 \text{ g betaxolol HCl/100 mL} = 0.28\%$$

5. An ophthalmic solution is prescribed to contain the equivalent of 0.3% of ciprofloxacin base (molecular weight, 332). How many milligrams of ciprofloxacin hydrochloride (molecular weight, 386) may be used to prepare each 5 mL of the solution?

$$\frac{0.3 \text{ g ciprofloxacin}}{100 \text{ mL}} \times \frac{1{,}000 \text{ mg}}{1 \text{ g}}$$
$$\times \frac{386 \text{ g/mole ciprofloxacin HCl}}{322 \text{ g/mole ciprofloxacin}} \times 5 \text{ mL}$$
$$= 17.44 \text{ mg ciprofloxacin HCl}$$

References

1. Ansel HC, Allen LV, Popovich NG. Pharmaceutical Dosage Forms and Drug Delivery Systems. 7th Ed. Baltimore, MD: Lippincott Williams & Wilkins, 1999:77–80.
2. The United States Pharmacopeia, 24th Rev., and National Formulary, 19th Ed. Rockville, MD: The United States Pharmacopeial Convention, 2000:2118– 2124.

19

SOME PHYSICAL CALCULATIONS

This chapter describes two types of physical calculations, specific gravity and thermometry. There are many additional physical calculations that pertain to pharmaceutics and formulations, which are described in other references and are not considered within the scope of this *Handbook*.

19.1 Specific Gravity

Definition. *Specific gravity* is a ratio, expressed decimally, of the weight of a substance to the weight of an equal volume of a standard substance at the same temperature.

Discussion. It is important to differentiate between *density* and specific gravity. Density is *mass per unit volume*; that is, the weight of a substance per unit of volume. For example, one milliliter of mercury weighs 13.6 g, and thus its density is *13.6 g/mL*. Whereas density is associated with units of weight and volume, specific gravity is an abstract number. Specific gravity describes the *relation* of the weight of a substance to that of a standard, such as water, which is the standard for most types of calculations in pharmacy and is assigned the specific gravity of 1.00. For comparison, the specific gravity of glycerin

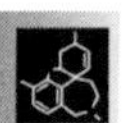

is 1.25, meaning that it is 1.25 times as heavy as an equivalent volume of water, and the specific gravity of alcohol is 0.81, meaning that it is 0.81 times as heavy as an equivalent volume of water.

- Substances that have a specific gravity of less than 1.00 are lighter than water.
- Substances that have a specific gravity greater than 1.00 are heavier than water.

Specific gravities are expressed decimally to as many places as the accuracy of their determination warrants. In general, two decimal places suffice. Specific gravities may be calculated, or they may be found for specific compounds in the *United States Pharmacopeia* (USP) or in other references.[2]

The specific gravity of a substance may be calculated, given its weight and volume, by the equation:

$$\text{Specific gravity (sp gr)} = \frac{\text{Weight of the substance (g)}}{\text{Weight of an equal volume of water (g)}}$$

In this equation, it is important to use the same unit of weight in both the numerator and denominator, generally grams, so that the units cancel out, leaving the quotient as an abstract number. It is also important to recognize that because 1 mL of water is considered to weigh 1 g, the "weight of an equal volume of water" in the denominator is the same numerical value in milliliters and grams. Thus, if 25 mL of a substance weighs 30 g, the "equal volume of water" (25 mL) weighs 25 g and the substance's specific gravity may be calculated as:

$$\text{sp gr} = \frac{30\text{ g}}{25\text{ g}} = 1.20$$

Knowing a substance's specific gravity, the weight of a given volume or the volume of a given weight may be de-

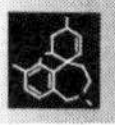

termined by using the above equation. For example, if a substance has a specific gravity of 0.80, the weight of 200 mL may be calculated as:

$$0.80 = \frac{x}{200\ g};\quad x = 160\ g$$

If a substance has a specific gravity of 1.20, the volume of 100 g may be calculated as:

$$1.20 = \frac{100\ g}{x};\quad x = 83.33\ g = 83.33\ mL$$

Key Point. Because water is the standard in specific gravity calculations and 1 mL of water is considered to weigh 1 g, the following equations may be used in calculating volume and weight:

$$mL \times sp\ gr = g$$

$$g \div sp\ gr = mL$$

Pharmacy Applications. Specific gravity is the enabling factor in converting quantities of substances in pharmaceutical formulas from weight to volume and vice versa. It is also used in calculations to convert expressions of strength in w/w, w/v, and v/v problems (see Chapter 4).

EXAMPLE PROBLEMS

1. If 150 mL of a sorbitol solution weighs 170 g, calculate its specific gravity.

$$\frac{170\ g}{150\ g} = 1.13$$

2. If 5 pints of diluted hydrochloric acid weighs 2.79 kg, calculate its specific gravity.

$$5 \text{ pt} \times \frac{473 \text{ mL}}{1 \text{ pint}} = 2{,}365 \text{ mL}$$

$$2.79 \text{ kg} = 2{,}790 \text{ g}$$

$$\frac{2{,}790 \text{ g}}{2{,}365 \text{ g}} = 1.18$$

3. Calculate the milliliters of polysorbate 80 (specific gravity, 1.08) required to prepare forty-eight 100-g tubes of the following formula for a progesterone vaginal cream.[1]

Progesterone, micronized	3 g
Polysorbate 80	1 g
Methylcellulose 2% gel	96 g

$$48 \text{ tubes} \times \frac{1 \text{ g polysorbate 80}}{1 \text{ tube}} = 48 \text{ g polysorbate 80}$$

$$\frac{48 \text{ g}}{1.08} = 44.44 \text{ mL}$$

4. If the following formula produces 50 glycerin suppositories, how many milliliters of glycerin (specific gravity, 1.25) would be used in the preparation of 96 suppositories?

Glycerin	91 g
Sodium stearate	9 g
Purified water	5 g

$$\frac{91 \text{ g}}{1.25} = 72.8 \text{ mL}$$

$$\frac{72.8 \text{ mL}}{50 \text{ suppositories}} \times 96 \text{ suppositories} = 139.78 \text{ mL}$$

5. Cocoa butter (theobroma oil) is solid at room temperature and has a specific gravity of 0.86. If a

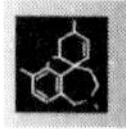

formula calls for 48 mL of theobroma oil, what would be its corresponding weight?

48 mL × 0.86 = 41.28 g

19.2 Thermometry

Thermometry is important in the use of controlled temperatures in chemical procedures, physical tests, and assays; in the proper storage of pharmaceuticals; and in the use of clinical thermometers in patient care. Both the centigrade, or Celsius, and the Fahrenheit scales for measuring temperature find application, and thus the pharmacist must be able to convert from one scale to the other.

Discussion. In 1709, the German scientist Gabriel Fahrenheit established a thermometer having a scale of 32° for the freezing point of water and 212° for its boiling point, a difference of 180° between these two points. In 1742, Anders Celsius, a Swedish astronomer, suggested the *centigrade thermometer* with a scale having 0° for the freezing point and 100° for the boiling point of water.

Because 100 centigrade degrees measure the same range of temperature as 180 Fahrenheit degrees, each centigrade degree is the equivalent of 1.8 or 9/5 of each Fahrenheit degree. This fact constitutes the basis for conversion between systems.

Although there are a number of different methods for conversion between the centigrade and Fahrenheit systems, the method described here is the one used in the USP[2]:

To convert °F to °C:

$$°C = \frac{5}{9} \times (°F - 32°)$$

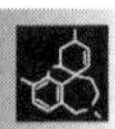

To convert °C to °F:

$$°F = \frac{9}{5} \times °C + 32°$$

EXAMPLE PROBLEMS

1. A low–reading thermometer used to diagnose hypothermia registers temperatures between 28.9°C and 42.2°C. Convert these temperatures to the Fahrenheit scale.

$$°F = \frac{9}{5} \times 28.9° + 32° = 84.02°$$

$$°F = \frac{9}{5} \times 42.2° + 32° = 107.96°$$

2. The USP expression "*excessive heat*" refers to any temperature above 104°F. Express this temperature on the centigrade scale.

$$°C = \frac{5}{9} \times (104° - 32°) = 40°$$

3. The USP defines a *refrigerator* as a cold place in which the temperature is maintained thermostatically between 2°C and 8°C. Express this temperature range on the Fahrenheit scale.

$$°F = \frac{9}{5} \times 2° + 32° = 35.6°$$

$$°F = \frac{9}{5} \times 8° + 32° = 46.4°$$

4. Cocoa butter melts between 30°C and 35°C. What is the range of its melting point on the Fahrenheit scale?

$$°F = \frac{9}{5} \times 30° + 32° = 86°$$

$$°F = \frac{9}{5} \times 35° + 32° = 95°$$

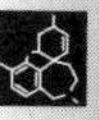

5. A woman charting her basal temperature finds that her body temperature ranged from 97.7°F to 98.6°F. Express these temperatures in degrees centigrade.

$$°C = \frac{5}{9} \times (97.7° - 32°) = 36.5°$$

$$°C = \frac{5}{9} \times (98.6° - 32°) = 37°$$

References

1. Allen LV Jr, ed. Progesterone 3% Vaginal Gel, International Journal of Pharmaceutical Compounding. 1998; 2:58.
2. The United States Pharmacopeia, 24th Rev., and National Formulary, 19th Ed. Rockville, MD: The United States Pharmacopeial Convention, 2000:2311.

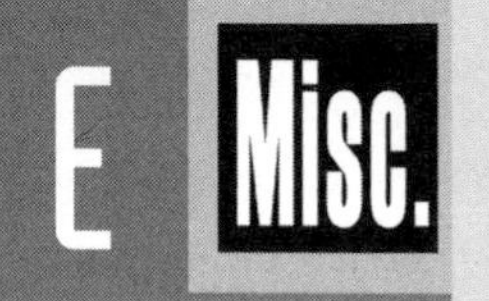

Miscellaneous Calculations

20

BASIC STATISTICAL CONCEPTS

Statistics may be defined as the science of the collection, classification, and interpretation of facts on the basis of relative number or occurrence as a ground for induction. Accordingly, all statistical studies begin with the gathering of reliable data. These data are then tabulated and analyzed for significance and validity by means of a number of mathematical and graphical procedures. This chapter presents an overview of statistics commonly used in pharmaceutical studies.

Although most pharmacists are not often called on to perform statistical calculations, statistical data are routinely encountered in the pharmaceutical literature. Therefore, it is important for pharmacists to understand the methods by which data are obtained, the basis for the application of various statistical tests, and the proper measures for the interpretation of the significance of test results. Such understanding also provides the underpinning to the use of computer programs for statistical analyses.

20.1 Measures of Central Tendency

A measure of central tendency is an aspect that deals with where on a scale the data are centered. The three

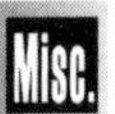

most common measures of central tendency are mean, median, and mode.

Definitions. The *mean*, also known as the *average*, is the total of the scores divided by the number of scores. The *median* is the value that lies in the middle of the data when the scores are arranged in numerical order, or the value that divides the distribution in half. The *mode* is simply the score that occurs the most often in the data set.

Expressions. Mean is usually represented by $\overline{X}$, median is sometimes abbreviated as Mdn, and mode is sometimes abbreviated as Mo. The units for all three measures correspond to the units of the values in the data set.

Discussion. To obtain the median or mode, the scores must be arranged in ascending order from lowest to highest (which is also known as an array). The median is then found by taking the middle value in an odd number of scores, or an average of the two middle values in an even number of scores. For example, using the following numbers as a data set arranged in ascending order:

1 4 6 8 13

the median would be the third value, or 6. If, however, the data set contained another value to generate an even number of scores as shown below:

1 4 6 8 13 15

the median would be the average of the third and fourth values, or $\frac{6 + 8}{2} = 7$.

After the data have been arranged in ascending order, the mode can be obtained as the value that occurs the most often. For example, using the data set shown below:

2 3 6 7 7 7 9 9 10

the mode would be 7 because it occurs three times and the other values occur only once or twice. In some data sets, more than one mode may exist if two values occur the same number of times and more than the other values. If the data set would have contained an additional value of 9, then the modes would have been 7 and 9 and the data would have been considered bimodal.

The mean is the measure of central tendency that is used by far the most often, and can be calculated using the following formula:

$$\overline{X} = \frac{\text{Sum of values (X)}}{\text{Number of values}} = \frac{\sum X}{n}$$

Using the first data set, the mean would be

$$\frac{1 + 4 + 6 + 8 + 13}{5} = \frac{32}{5} = 6.4$$

When the scores in a set of data are multiplied or divided by a constant, the mean will also be multiplied or divided by that same constant. If a constant is added to or subtracted from the data, the constant is also added to or subtracted from the mean. For instance, if all of the scores in the previous data set are multiplied by two, then the mean would be $6.4 \times 2 = 12.8$. To prove this point, the mean of the data can be recalculated as follows:

$$(1 \quad 4 \quad 6 \quad 8 \quad 13) \times 2 = 2 \quad 8 \quad 12 \quad 16 \quad 26$$

$$\frac{2 + 8 + 12 + 16 + 26}{5} = 12.8$$

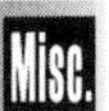

The mean has the advantage that it can be calculated using a formula and that the data do not first have to be arranged in any particular order before the mean can be calculated, unlike the median and mode. However, the mean is affected by "extreme" scores, sometimes referred to as "outliers," that may cause the mean to be an inaccurate measure of central tendency in some data sets. The median and mode have the advantage that they are not affected by these extreme scores. The following data set, as shown previously, can be used to demonstrate this point:

2 3 6 7 7 7 9 9 10

mode = 7, median (5th value) = 7, and mean = 60/9 = 6.67

If the data contained an additional score of 72, the values would be affected as follows:

mode = 7, median (5th and 6th values) = 7, and mean = 132/10 = 13.2

Key Points. Because the most commonly used measure of central tendency is the mean, care should be taken to ensure that the mean accurately represents the data and is not skewed by extreme scores.

Pharmacy Applications. In most reports on pharmaceutical research, whether it is a journal article or a package insert, the data are summarized using measures of central tendency rather than presented as raw data that would be confusing to the reader. Also, a measure of central tendency can indicate the accuracy of a given set of data if a target value is known (e.g., the mean amount of drug in a batch of tablets labeled to contain

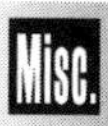

250 mg of drug is 244.87 mg). The observer can then draw conclusions as to the accuracy of a certain set of data.

EXAMPLE PROBLEMS

1. An independent pharmacy owner decided to record the number of prescriptions filled during a 1-week period to determine staffing requirements. He recorded the following results:

Monday: 215 prescriptions

Tuesday: 95 prescriptions

Wednesday: 110 prescriptions

Thursday: 89 prescriptions

Friday: 95 prescriptions

Saturday: 156 prescriptions

Sunday: closed

Determine the mean, median, and mode for this data set.

$$\bar{X} = \frac{215 + 95 + 110 + 89 + 95 + 156}{6} = \frac{760}{6}$$

$$= 126.67 \text{ prescriptions}$$

Arranged in ascending order:

89 95 95 110 156 215

$$\text{Median} = \frac{95 + 110}{2} = 102.5 \text{ prescriptions}$$

Mode = 95 prescriptions

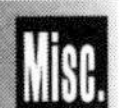

2. Ten pharmacy students were asked how many hours that they studied in preparation for a Medicinal Chemistry exam. The results were as follows:

Student	Number of Hours Spent Studying
1	12
2	4
3	8
4	2
5	6
6	8
7	11
8	6
9	4
10	8

What are the median, mode, and mean for this data set?

Arranged in ascending order:

2 4 4 6 6 8 8 8 11 12

$$\text{Median} = \frac{6 + 8}{2} = 7 \text{ hours}$$

Mode = 8 hours$\bar{X}$

$$\bar{X} = \frac{2 + 4 + 4 + 6 + 6 + 8 + 8 + 8 + 11 + 12}{10}$$

$$= 6.9 \text{ hours}$$

20.2 Measures of Variation

Measures of variation indicate the degree to which the individual scores are clustered near, or deviate from, the measure of central tendency. In essence, measures of variation are used in conjunction with measures of central tendency to more accurately represent the data. There are many measures of variation, but range, average deviation, standard deviation, and coefficient of variation will be discussed here.

Definitions. *Range* is simply the difference between the largest and smallest scores in a data set. *Deviation* is the amount by which a given score differs from the mean of the data set and is represented as $(X - \bar{X})$. Another measure of central tendency, median or mode, can be substituted for the mean in the calculation of deviation, but this is not commonly used. Notice that in the determination of the deviation, the value can be a positive or negative number. In some cases, the absolute value of the deviation is used, meaning that the algebraic sign is dropped from the negative numbers and is shown mathematically using straight brackets (e.g., $|-4| = 4$). The term absolute deviation refers to the absolute value of the deviation and is often abbreviated using the letter *d*. The *average deviation*, sometimes referred to as *mean absolute deviation*, is the mean of the absolute deviations. The *standard deviation* is the square root of the sum of the squared deviations divided by the number of scores minus one. *Coefficient of variation*, also known as *relative standard deviation*, is the standard deviation of a sample divided by its mean.

Expressions. With the exception of coefficient of variation, the units on the measures of variation correspond to the units of the scores in the data set. Coefficient of variation, usually abbreviated as CV or RSD, has no units or may be multiplied by 100 and expressed as a percent. Range is often represented by R, and average deviation is often shortened to AD. Standard deviation has several representations, but the ones most commonly seen are σ, s, or SD.

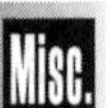

Discussion. The following example data set, as seen in the previous section, will be used throughout this discussion:

1 4 6 8 13

The range for these data would be 13 − 1 = 12. To calculate the average and standard deviation, the deviation and squared deviation of each score must first be calculated using the mean of 6.4 in the following manner:

Score	Deviation	Absolute Deviation	Deviation Squared
1	$1 - 6.4 = -5.4$	5.4	$(-5.4)^2 = 29.16$
4	$4 - 6.4 = -2.4$	2.4	$(-2.4)^2 = 5.76$
6	$6 - 6.4 = -0.4$	0.4	$(-0.4)^2 = 0.16$
8	$8 - 6.4 = 1.6$	1.6	$(1.6)^2 = 2.56$
13	$13 - 6.4 = 6.6$	6.6	$(6.6)^2 = 43.56$

The absolute deviation is calculated as follows:

$$AD = \frac{\Sigma|X - \overline{X}|}{n} = \frac{\Sigma d}{n}$$

$$= \frac{5.4 + 2.4 + 0.4 + 1.6 + 6.6}{5} = \frac{16.4}{5} = 3.28$$

The standard deviation is calculated using the following equation:

$$\sigma = \sqrt{\frac{\Sigma(X - \overline{X})^2}{n - 1}} = \sqrt{\frac{\Sigma d^2}{n - 1}}$$

$$= \sqrt{\frac{29.16 + 5.76 + 0.16 + 2.56 + 43.56}{5 - 1}}$$

$$= \sqrt{\frac{81.2}{4}} = 4.51$$

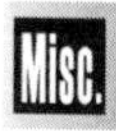

Finally, the coefficient of variation is calculated as follows:

$$CV = \frac{\sigma}{\overline{X}} = \frac{4.51}{6.4} = 0.705 \text{ or } 70.5\%$$

Standard deviation is the most often used measurement of variation because it is easily correlated to most data sets by the evidence that approximately 67% of the scores fall within one standard deviation of the mean, and approximately 95% of the scores fall within two standard deviations of the mean. For example, a certain batch of 100 tablets is reported to contain a mean drug amount of 244.87 mg with a standard deviation of 3.45 mg (commonly reported as 244.87 ± 3.45 mg). Using this information, it can be estimated that 67 tablets will contain between 241.42 mg (244.87 mg − 3.45 mg) and 248.32 mg (244.87 mg + 3.45 mg) of drug, and 95 tablets will contain between 237.97 mg (244.87 mg − 2 × 3.45 mg) and 251.77 mg (244.87 mg + 2 × 3.45 mg) of drug. When the scores in a set of data are multiplied or divided by a constant, the standard deviation will also be multiplied or divided by that same constant. However, if a constant is added to or subtracted from the data, the standard deviation remains unchanged.

Key Points. Measures of variation are used in conjunction with measures of central tendency to represent the "complete picture" of the data. The smaller the value for the measure of variation, the closer the data fall to the mean or other measure of central tendency.

Pharmacy Applications. Just as a measure of central tendency is used to summarize raw data, measures of variation are used to indicate the precision of a set of data. For example, two batches of 100 tablets labeled to

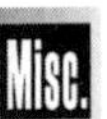

contain 250 mg of drug are reported with the following means and standard deviations:

Batch 1: 244.87 ± 3.45 mg
Batch 2: 248.55 ± 19.32 mg

Although the mean of the second batch is closer to the target value of 250 mg, the data are not as precise because approximately 67 tablets contain between 229.23 and 267.87 mg of drug, as compared with a range of 241.42 to 248.32 mg for Batch 1.

EXAMPLE PROBLEMS

1. Calculate the range, average deviation, standard deviation, and coefficient of variation for the data presented in Example Problem 1 in the previous section.

Range = 215 − 89 = 126 prescriptions

Number of ℞	Absolute Deviations (d)	d^2
215	$\lvert 215 - 126.67 \rvert = 88.33$	7,802.19
95	$\lvert 95 - 126.67 \rvert = 31.67$	1,002.99
110	$\lvert 110 - 126.67 \rvert = 16.67$	277.89
89	$\lvert 89 - 126.67 \rvert = 37.67$	1,419.03
95	$\lvert 95 - 126.67 \rvert = 31.67$	1,002.99
156	$\lvert 156 - 126.67 \rvert = 29.33$	860.25
Total	235.34	12,365.34

$$AD = \frac{235.34}{6} = 39.22 \text{ prescriptions}$$

$$\sigma = \sqrt{\frac{12{,}365.34}{6 - 1}} = \sqrt{2{,}473.07}$$

$$= 49.73 \text{ prescriptions}$$

$$CV = \frac{49.73}{126.67} = 0.39$$

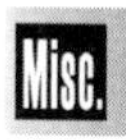

2. Caregivers at two different extended-care facilities were asked to measure a 2-teaspoonful dose of syrup using whatever measuring device he or she wished to use. Each caregiver measured the dose, then it was weighed and divided by the specific gravity of the syrup to determine the exact amount measured. The amounts measured were recorded as shown. Use this information to answer the questions below.

Group A	Group B
11.2 mL	9.5 mL
14 mL	7.1 mL
8.9 mL	10.6 mL

A. Calculate the mean and standard deviation for each group.

Group A	d	d^2	Group B	d	d^2
11.2 mL	0.17	0.028	9.5 mL	0.43	0.19
14 mL	2.63	6.93	7.1 mL	1.97	3.87
8.9 mL	2.47	6.08	10.6 mL	1.53	2.35
Totals:					
34.1 mL		13.05	27.2 mL		6.41

$$\overline{X}_A = \frac{34.1 \text{ mL}}{3} = 11.37 \text{ mL}$$

$$\sigma_A = \sqrt{\frac{13.05}{2}} = 2.55 \text{ mL}$$

$$\overline{X}_B = \frac{27.2 \text{ mL}}{3} = 9.07 \text{ mL}$$

$$\sigma_B = \sqrt{\frac{6.41}{2}} = 1.79 \text{ mL}$$

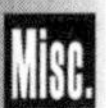

B. Which group is more accurate in their measurement? Why?

Group B is more accurate because the mean is closer to the target value of 10 mL than the mean for Group A.

C. Which group is more precise in their measurement? Why?

Group B is more precise because the standard deviation is smaller than the standard deviation for Group A.

D. Calculate the coefficient of variation for each group.

$$CV_A = \frac{2.55}{11.37} = 0.225$$

$$CV_B = \frac{1.79}{9.07} = 0.197$$

20.3 Statistical Tests

Statistics are used to determine whether or not research findings are significant at a certain level, and myriad statistical tests exist for this purpose. The appropriate statistical test to be used is determined by the type of data collected, number of study groups, sample size within each group, and research study design. Furthermore, statistical tests are based on sample populations that should predict the behavior of the whole population. Regardless of the statistical test used, a *P value* will be generated, which is usually reported with the research results, and the discussion in this section will focus on that topic. The intent of this section is to equip the pharmacist with the basic knowledge for evaluating statistical results, but not for proposing his or her own statistical design for a research project.

Definitions. The *null hypothesis* states that the treatment being studied has no effect, and the *research*, or *alternative*, *hypothesis* states that the treatment does have an effect. The *P value* is the probability of the observed difference between research groups occurring if the null hypothesis is true. Or, more simply stated, the *P* value is the probability that the difference observed between two or more groups is insignificant.

Discussion. In most areas of research a *P* value of less than .05 is considered to be acceptable, which means that if the calculated *P* value is less than .05, the null hypothesis will be rejected. The *P* value reflects the degree of certainty that the conclusions drawn from the study are correct. For the purpose of this discussion, consider the following scenario:

> A pharmaceutical company has developed a new drug for the treatment of hyperlipidemia, and the researchers have chosen to compare it with another antihyperlipidemic drug available on the market. Group A will receive the investigational drug for 16 weeks, and Group B will receive the current prescription drug. The patients will be randomly assigned to these groups and will also adhere to the same strict diet. Cholesterol levels will be assessed for patients in both groups at the beginning and end of the 16-week study period. Results will be reported as percent decrease in total cholesterol.

The null hypothesis for this study is that both groups will have the same percent decrease in total cholesterol. The research hypothesis for this study is that both groups will not have the same percent decrease in total cholesterol, and from the viewpoint of the pharmaceutical company, the difference should show that Group A

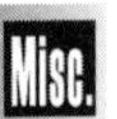

will have a larger percent decrease in cholesterol than Group B.

If the data are analyzed by a statistical test, such as an unpaired *t*-test, and a *P* value of .028 is calculated, the researchers can reject the null hypothesis. The *P* value of .028 indicates that the probability of incorrectly rejecting the null hypothesis is 2.8%, or that the researchers can be 97.2% certain that treatment with the new drug does have a *different* effect than treatment with the older drug. A summary of the data (e.g., mean and standard deviation) must be examined to determine whether the effect of the new drug is greater or less than that of the older drug.

If, however, a *P* value of .118 is calculated from an appropriate statistical test, the null hypothesis will be accepted, or the conclusion will be drawn that the new drug and the older drug both lower cholesterol to the same extent. The researchers can only be 88.2% certain that treatment with the new drug produces a different effect than treatment with the older drug, which is generally considered to be an unacceptable probability.

Key Points. The lower the *P* value, the greater the degree of certainty that the results for various groups are not the same. The actual data or data summaries must be examined to determine what the difference truly indicates.

Pharmacy Applications. The pharmacist should beware of the overuse of terms such as "statistically significant." A *P* value of less than .05 merely indicates that a difference is observed, and the clinical implications of that difference must be considered.

F

Competency Assessment

F. COMPETENCY ASSESSMENT

Answers to the following problems appear at the end of this section, beginning on page 295.

1. Atrovent nasal spray contains 0.06% ipratropium bromide. If each depression of the valve delivers a 42-μg dose of the drug, how many doses are contained in a 15-mL container?

2. ℞

Tetracycline HCl	0.85%
Tetracaine HCl	0.65%
Dextrose (to make isotonic)	q.s.
Purified water q.s.	30 mL

How much of each ingredient would be needed to fill this prescription? (NaCl equivalents: tetracycline HCl = 0.12, tetracaine HCl = 0.18, dextrose = 0.18)

3. The dose of a drug is 35 mg/kg/day. What would be the infusion rate (mL/hr) of a 0.4% solution of the drug if administered to a patient weighing 138 lb?

4. Use the following patient information to answer the questions below:

NAME: Jane Doe		PATIENT NUMBER: 1225	
DATE OF ADMIT: 8-30-02		ALLERGIES: Codeine	SEX: F
HEIGHT: 5′6″	WEIGHT: 110 lb	AGE: 45 yr	
DIAGNOSIS: Malnutrition secondary to Crohn's disease			
PERTINENT LAB VALUES: Na = 122, K = 5.1, glucose = 72, serum creatinine = 0.8			

A. Calculate the ideal body weight, body mass index, lean body mass, body surface area, creatinine clearance, resting metabolic energy, and total daily calories (activity factor = 1.3) for this patient.
B. Calculate the parenteral nutrition and fluid requirements for this patient.
C. How many milliliters each of a 7% amino acid solution, 50% dextrose solution, and 20% lipid emulsion would be needed to supply the daily caloric needs for this patient?

5. The adult dose of doxorubicin is 60 to 75 mg/m^2 given as a single intravenous injection. What would be the dosage range of doxorubicin for a patient who is 5′3″ tall and weighs 142 lb?

6. You have a prescription formula to prepare that requires 8 mg of drug. Using starch as the diluent, how would you obtain this quantity on a balance with a sensitivity of 2 mg and with an accuracy of ±5%?

7. What would be the osmolarity of a D5NS solution? (molecular weight of dextrose = 180, molecular weight of NaCl = 58.5, assume complete dissociation)

8. If the solution in Question 7 is infused at a rate of 32 gtts/min using an administration set with a drop

factor of 20 gtts/mL, how many milliequivalents of sodium is the patient receiving per day?

9. A formula for a transdermal analgesic gel is as follows[1,2]:

℞		
	Ketoprofen	10 g
	Cyclobenzaprine HCl	1 g
	Lidocaine	5 g
	Sorbic acid	0.2 g
	Poloxamer lecithin organogel	83.8 g

A. You first need to determine the specific gravity of this gel, and you find that 12 mL of the gel weighs 10.85 g. What is the specific gravity of this gel? (NOTE: These numbers are hypothetical and should not be used for actual dose determination.)

B. You want to deliver this gel using a syringe; therefore, you need to determine the dose measured by volume. What would be the dose of this gel (in milliliters) to deliver 100 mg of ketoprofen?

C. How many milligrams each of cyclobenzaprine HCl and lidocaine would be delivered with this dose?

10. Drug A has a minimum effective concentration of 0.5 mg /dL and a minimum toxic concentration of 8.1 mg /dL. Drug B has a minimum effective concentration of 7.3 mg /dL and a minimum toxic concentration of 12.6 mg /dL. Which drug is safer, and why?

11. How many milligrams of fluocinonide should be added to 15 g of an ointment containing 0.05% w/w to increase the strength to 0.08% w/w?

12. Rum-K liquid contains 15% potassium chloride. How many milliequivalents of potassium are contained in each teaspoonful dose? (molecular weight of K = 39, molecular weight of Cl = 35.5)

13. The following is a formula for an athletic-analgesic rub[3]:

℞		
	Capsaicin	50 mg
	Methyl salicylate	20 g
	Menthol	2 g
	Camphor	5 g
	Xanthan gum	500 mg
	Olive oil	25 mL
	Purified water q.s.	100 mL

How much of each ingredient will be needed to prepare one pint of this formulation?

14. A patient has been receiving 20 mg of a drug daily by intravenous infusion while in the hospital; however, to leave the hospital, the patient needs to switch to the oral dosage form of the drug, which is 39% bioavailable. The drug is available in 5-, 10-, 25-, and 50-mg tablets and should be given twice daily. Calculate an oral dosage regimen for this patient.

15. A pharmacist needs to prepare 36 mL of a 0.2% dexamethasone solution for iontophoresis. How many milliliters of an injection containing dexamethasone sodium phosphate equivalent to 4 mg of dexamethasone per milliliter will be needed to prepare this solution?

16.

℞		
	Clindamycin	0.5 g
	Propylene glycol	6 mL
	Purified water	8 mL
	Isopropyl alcohol q.s.	60 mL

A. How many capsules, each containing clindamycin hydrochloride equivalent to 150 mg of clindamycin, would be used in preparing the prescription?

B. If the contents of each capsule weigh 310 mg, how many milligrams of the powder from the opened capsules would you need to weigh to prepare the prescription?

C. What would be the percent strength (w/v) of clindamycin hydrochloride in the solution? (800 μg clindamycin = 1 mg clindamycin HCl)

17. At 7:00 PM, you receive an order in the hospital pharmacy that says "Increase IV fluids to 100 mL/hr." When you check the patient's profile, you find that she was receiving Lactated Ringer's Injection 1,000 mL at a rate of 75 mL/hr and that the last container was started at 12:30 PM. When should the next container of solution be started, assuming that the flow rate on the existing container was changed at 7:00 PM?

18. Paregoric is 4% v/v opium tincture that contains 10% w/v opium. If opium contains 10% w/w morphine, how many milligrams of morphine are contained in a 2-fl oz bottle of paregoric?

19. A clinical pharmacist receives the following patient information sheet:

NAME: Christopher Smith	PATIENT NUMBER: 11194	
DATE OF ADMIT: 8-30-02	ALLERGIES: Penicillin	SEX: M
HEIGHT: 2′4″	WEIGHT: 29 lb	AGE: 4 yr

The pediatrician writes an order for enalapril for Chris and gives instructions for the pharmacist to calculate an appropriate dose. The adult dose for enalapril is 10 mg daily. What should be the dose for this patient?

20. ℞ Codeine phosphate 15 mg /tsp
Elixophyllin elixir 100 mL
Robitussin syrup ad 180 mL
Sig: ʒi q8h

The concentration of theophylline in Elixophyllin elixir is 80 mg/15 mL. How many milligrams of theophylline would be taken daily?

21. The following is an order for a hyperalimentation solution:

Order	Component Source
Amino acids 3%	500 mL of 8.5% amino acids injection
Dextrose 15%	500 mL of 50% dextrose injection
Sodium chloride 20 mEq	50-mL vial of 14.6% solution
Potassium chloride 25 mEq	25-mL vial of 14.9% solution
Magnesium sulfate 8 mEq	10-mL vial of 50% magnesium sulfate heptahydrate solution
Calcium gluconate 10 mEq	50-mL vial of 10% solution
Potassium phosphate 15 mmol	10-mL vial of 3 mmol/mLsolution
Sterile water for injection to make 1,000 mL	1,000 mL of sterile water for injection

What volume of each ingredient would be needed to prepare this solution? (Assume volumes are additive; molecular weight of NaCl = 58.5, molecular weight of KCl = 74.5, molecular weight of $MgSO_4 \cdot 7H_2O$ = 246, molecular weight of $Ca(C_6H_{11}O_7)_2$ = 430)

22. Concentrated hydrochloric acid is a 38% w/w solution of HCl in water and has a specific gravity of 1.18. How many milliliters of concentrated hydrochloric acid are needed to prepare 1 quart of a 1:200 w/v HCl solution?

23. The following is a formula for coal tar ointment:

Coal tar	2 parts
Polysorbate 80	1 part
Zinc oxide paste	197 parts

How many grams of each ingredient are required to prepare 120 g of coal tar ointment?

24. A compounding pharmacist prepares a batch of 100 capsules. A sample of 10 capsules is weighed with the following results:

210 mg	205 mg
185 mg	195 mg
200 mg	210 mg
190 mg	200 mg
225 mg	190 mg

Calculate the mean and standard deviation for these data.

25. You need to prepare nystatin troches containing 400,000 units per troche.

A. How many troches can be prepared from 2 oz of nystatin powder? (1 mg nystatin = 4400 units)

B. The melting point of the base used to prepare these troches is approximately 45°C. What is this temperature in degrees Fahrenheit?

Answers to Problems

1. $$\frac{1 \text{ dose}}{42\ \mu g} \times \frac{1 \times 10^6\ \mu g}{1 \text{ g}} \times \frac{0.06 \text{ g}}{100 \text{ mL}} \times 15 \text{ mL}$$
$$= 214.29 \text{ doses} \approx 214 \text{ doses}$$

2. $$\frac{0.9 \text{ g}}{100 \text{ mL}} \times 30 \text{ mL} \times \frac{1{,}000 \text{ mg}}{1 \text{ g}} = 270 \text{ mg of NaCl}$$

in 30 mL of an isotonic solution

Tetracycline HCl:

$$\frac{0.85\text{ g}}{100\text{ mL}} \times 30\text{ mL} \times \frac{1{,}000\text{ mg}}{1\text{ g}} = 255\text{ mg}$$

Tetracaine HCl:

$$\frac{0.65\text{ g}}{100\text{ mL}} \times 30\text{ mL} \times \frac{1{,}000\text{ mg}}{1\text{ g}} = 195\text{ mg}$$

Sodium chloride equivalents:

$$(255\text{ mg} \times 0.12) + (195\text{ mg} \times 0.18) = 65.7\text{ mg}$$

Sodium chloride: $270\text{ mg} - 65.7\text{ mg} = 204.3\text{ mg}$

Dextrose: $\dfrac{204.3\text{ mg}}{0.18} = 1{,}135\text{ mg}$

Purified water: q.s. 30 mL

3. $\dfrac{35\text{ mg}}{1\text{ kg/day}} \times \dfrac{1\text{ kg}}{2.2\text{ lb}} \times 138\text{ lb} = 2{,}195.45\text{ mg/day}$

$$\frac{2{,}195.45\text{ mg}}{1\text{ day}} \times \frac{1\text{ g}}{1{,}000\text{ mg}} \times \frac{100\text{ mL}}{0.4\text{ g}} \times \frac{1\text{ day}}{24\text{ hr}} = 22.87\text{ mL/hr} \approx 23\text{ mL/hr}$$

4. A. $110\text{ lb} \times \dfrac{1\text{ kg}}{2.2\text{ lb}} = 50\text{ kg}$

$5'6'' = 66''$

$$66\text{ in} \times \frac{2.54\text{ cm}}{1\text{ in}} = 167.64\text{ cm}$$

$$\times \frac{1\text{ m}}{100\text{ cm}} = 1.68\text{ m}$$

$$\text{IBW} = 45.5\text{ kg} + 2.3\text{ kg} \times 6\text{ in} = 59.3\text{ kg}$$

$$\text{BMI} = \frac{50\text{ kg}}{(1.68\text{ m})^2} = 17.79$$

$$\text{LBM} = [1.07 \times 50 \text{ kg}] - 148\left\{\frac{[50 \text{ kg}]^2}{[100 \times 1.68 \text{ m}]^2}\right\} = 40.33 \text{ kg}$$

$$\text{BSA} = \sqrt{\frac{167.64 \text{ cm} \times 50 \text{ kg}}{3{,}600}} = \sqrt{2.33} = 1.53 \text{ m}^2$$

$$\text{CrCl} = 0.85 \times \frac{(140 - 45 \text{ yr}) \times 50 \text{ kg}}{72 \times 0.8 \text{ mg/dL}} = 70.1 \text{ mL/min}$$

$$\text{RME} = 655 + (9.6 \times 50 \text{ kg}) + (1.8 \times 167.64 \text{ cm}) - (4.7 \times 45 \text{ yr}) = 1{,}225.25 \text{ kcal/day}$$

$$\text{TDC} = 1{,}225.25 \text{ kcal/day} \times 1.3 = 1{,}592.83 \text{ kcal/day}$$

B. Protein: $50 \text{ kg} \times \frac{0.8\text{g}}{1 \text{ kg/day}} = 40 \text{ g/day}$

$$\frac{40 \text{ g}}{1 \text{ day}} \times \frac{4 \text{ kcal}}{1 \text{ g}} = 160 \text{ kcal/day}$$

Using an average lipid requirement of 35% of total daily calories and assuming that 20% lipid emulsion will be used:

$$1{,}592.83 \text{ kcal/day} \times 35\% = 557.49 \text{ kcal/day from lipid emulsion}$$

Lipids: $\frac{557.49 \text{ kcal}}{1 \text{ day}} \times \frac{1 \text{ g}}{10 \text{ kcal}} = 55.75 \text{ g/day}$

$$1{,}592.83 \text{ kcal/day} - 160 \text{ kcal/day} - 557.49 \text{ kcal/day} = 875.34 \text{ kcal/day}$$

Dextrose:

$$\frac{875.34 \text{ kcal}}{1 \text{ day}} \times \frac{1 \text{ g}}{3.4 \text{ kcal}} = 257.45 \text{ g/day}$$

Fluid: $50 \text{ kg} \times \frac{30 \text{ mL}}{1 \text{ kg/day}} = 1{,}500 \text{ mL/day}$

Fluid:

$$\frac{1{,}592.83 \text{ kcal}}{1 \text{ day}} \times \frac{1 \text{ mL}}{1 \text{ kcal}} = 1{,}592.83 \text{ mL/day}$$

The patient should receive 40 g of protein, 55.75 g of lipids, 257.45 g of dextrose, and 1,500 to 1,592.83 mL of fluid per day.

C. Amino acids: $40 \text{ g} \times \frac{100 \text{ mL}}{7 \text{ g}} = 571.43 \text{ mL}$

Dextrose: $257.45 \text{ g} \times \frac{100 \text{ mL}}{50 \text{ g}} = 514.9 \text{ mL}$

Lipids: $55.75 \text{ g} \times \frac{100 \text{ mL}}{20 \text{ g}} = 278.74 \text{ mL}$

5. $5'3'' = 63''$

BSA (from nomogram in Appendix C) = 1.67 m^2

$$\frac{60 \text{ mg}}{1 \text{ m}^2} \times 1.67 \text{ m}^2 = 100.2 \text{ mg}$$

$$\frac{75 \text{ mg}}{1 \text{ m}^2} \times 1.67 \text{ m}^2 = 125.25 \text{ mg}$$

Dosage range: 100.2–125.25 mg

6. Least weighable quantity: $\frac{100\% \times 2 \text{ mg}}{5\%} = 40 \text{ mg}$

Multiple factor selected: 5
Aliquot portion selected: 40 mg

Weigh (5×8 mg)	40 mg (drug)
Dilute with	160 mg (starch)
to make (5×40 mg)	200 mg (mixture)

Weigh 1/5 of dilution, $\frac{200 \text{ mg}}{5} = 40$ mg, which contains 8 mg of drug.

7. $$\frac{5 \text{ g}}{100 \text{ mL}} \times \frac{1{,}000 \text{ mg}}{1 \text{ g}} \times \frac{1 \text{ mOsmol}}{180 \text{ mg}} \times \frac{1{,}000 \text{ mL}}{1 \text{ L}} = 277.78 \text{ mOsmol/L}$$

$$\frac{0.9 \text{ g}}{100 \text{ mL}} \times \frac{1{,}000 \text{ mg}}{1 \text{ g}} \times \frac{2 \text{ mOsmol}}{58.5 \text{ mg}} \times \frac{1{,}000 \text{ mL}}{1 \text{ L}} = 307.69 \text{ mOsmol/L}$$

$$\text{Total} = 277.78 \text{ mOsmol/L} + 307.69 \text{ mOsmol/L} = 585.47 \text{ mOsmol/L}$$

8. $$\frac{0.9 \text{ g}}{100 \text{ mL}} \times \frac{1{,}000 \text{ mg}}{1 \text{ g}} \times \frac{1 \text{ mEq}}{58.5 \text{ mg}} = 0.15 \text{ mEq/mL}$$

$$\frac{0.15 \text{ mEq}}{1 \text{ mL}} \times \frac{1 \text{ mL}}{20 \text{ gtts}} \times \frac{32 \text{ gtts}}{1 \text{ min}} \times \frac{60 \text{ min}}{1 \text{ hr}} \times \frac{24 \text{ hr}}{1 \text{ day}} = 354.46 \text{ mEq/day}$$

9. A. $$\text{specific gravity} = \frac{10.85 \text{ g}}{12 \text{ g}} = 0.904$$

B. Total weight of gel:
$10 \text{ g} + 1 \text{ g} + 5 \text{ g} + 0.2 \text{ g} + 83.8 \text{ g} = 100 \text{ g}$

100 g of gel contains 10 g of ketoprofen

$$\frac{100 \text{ g gel}}{10 \text{ g ketoprofen}} \times \frac{1 \text{ g}}{1{,}000 \text{ mg}}$$

$$\times \frac{100 \text{ mg ketoprofen}}{1 \text{ dose}} = 1 \text{ g gel/dose}$$

$$\frac{1 \text{ g gel/dose}}{0.904} = 1.11 \text{ mL/dose}$$

C. $\frac{1 \text{ g gel}}{1 \text{ dose}} \times \frac{1 \text{ g cyclobenzaprine HCl}}{100 \text{ g gel}}$

$$\times \frac{1{,}000 \text{ mg}}{1 \text{ g}} = 10 \text{ mg cyclobenzaprine HCl}$$

$$\frac{1 \text{ g gel}}{1 \text{ dose}} \times \frac{5 \text{ g lidocaine}}{100 \text{ g gel}} \times \frac{1{,}000 \text{ mg}}{1 \text{ g}}$$

$$= 50 \text{ mg lidocaine}$$

10. Therapeutic window A =
8.1 mg/dL − 0.5 mg/dL = 7.6 mg/dL

Therapeutic window B =
12.6 mg/dL − 7.3 mg/dL = 5.3 mg/dL

Drug A is safer because it has a larger therapeutic window.

11.

100%		0.03
	0.08%	
0.05%		99.92

Relative amounts = 0.03:99.92

$$\frac{0.03 \text{ parts fluocinonide}}{99.92 \text{ parts } 0.05\% \text{ ointment}} = \frac{x}{15 \text{ g}}$$

$$x = 0.0045 \text{ g} \times \frac{1{,}000 \text{ mg}}{1 \text{ g}} = 4.5 \text{ mg}$$

12. $$\frac{15\text{ g}}{100\text{ mL}} \times \frac{5\text{ mL}}{1\text{ tsp}} \times \frac{1\text{ tsp}}{1\text{ dose}} \times \frac{1{,}000\text{ mg}}{1\text{ g}} \times \frac{1\text{ mEq}}{74.5\text{ mg}} = 10.07\text{ mEq/dose}$$

13. 1 pint = 473 mL

Capsaicin: $\frac{50\text{ mg}}{100\text{ mL}} \times 473\text{ mL} = 236.5\text{ mg}$

Methyl salicylate: $\frac{20\text{ g}}{100\text{ mL}} \times 473\text{ mL} = 94.6\text{ g}$

Menthol: $\frac{2\text{ g}}{100\text{ mL}} \times 473\text{ mL} = 9.46\text{ g}$

Camphor: $\frac{5\text{ g}}{100\text{ mL}} \times 473\text{ mL} = 23.65\text{ g}$

Xanthan gum:

$$\frac{500\text{ mg}}{100\text{ mL}} \times \frac{1\text{ g}}{1{,}000\text{ mg}} \times 473\text{ mL} = 2.37\text{ g}$$

Olive oil: $\frac{25\text{ mL}}{100\text{ mL}} \times 473\text{ mL} = 118.25\text{ mL}$

Purified water: q.s. 473 mL

14. F for the IV route is 1 or 100%

$100\% \times 20\text{ mg/day} = 39\% \times \text{Dose}_{oral}$

$\text{Dose}_{oral} = 51.28\text{ mg/day}$

$$\frac{51.28\text{ mg}}{1\text{ day}} \times \frac{1\text{ day}}{2\text{ doses}} = 25.64\text{ mg/dose}$$

The patient should take one 25-mg tablet twice daily.

15. $\frac{0.2\text{ g}}{100\text{ mL solution}} \times 36\text{ mL solution} \times \frac{1{,}000\text{ mg}}{1\text{ g}} \times \frac{1\text{ mL injection}}{4\text{ mg}} = 18\text{ mL of the injection}$

16. A. $0.5\text{ g} \times \frac{1{,}000\text{ mg}}{1\text{ g}} \times \frac{1\text{ capsule}}{150\text{ mg}} = 3.33\text{ capsules}$

The prescription requires 3.33 capsules, but measuring one-third of a capsule is impractical. Therefore, 4 capsules would be used and the contents weighed as in Part B below.

B. $0.5\text{ g clindamycin} \times \frac{1{,}000\text{ mg}}{1\text{ g}} \times \frac{310\text{ mg powder}}{150\text{ mg clindamycin}} = 1{,}033.33\text{ mg powder}$

C. $\frac{0.5\text{ g clindamycin}}{60\text{ mL}} \times \frac{1 \times 10^{6}\ \mu\text{g}}{1\text{ g}} \times \frac{1\text{ mg clindamycin HCl}}{800\ \mu\text{g clindamycin}} \times \frac{1\text{ g}}{1{,}000\text{ mg}} \times 100 = 1.04\%$

17. 12:30 PM to 7:00 PM = 6.5 hours

$\frac{75\text{ mL}}{1\text{ hr}} \times 6.5\text{ hr} = 487.5\text{ mL infused}$

$1{,}000\text{ mL} - 487.5\text{ mL} = 512.5\text{ mL remaining}$

$512.5\text{ mL} \times \frac{1\text{ hr}}{100\text{ mL}} = 5.13\text{ hr} \approx 5\text{ hr}$

7:00 PM + 5 hr = 12:00 AM

18. $2\text{ oz paregoric} \times \frac{29.57\text{ mL}}{1\text{ oz}} \times \frac{4\text{ mL opium tincture}}{100\text{ mL paregoric}} = 2.37\text{ mL opium tincture}$

$$2.37 \text{ mL opium tincture} \times \frac{10 \text{ g opium}}{100 \text{ mL opium tincture}} = 0.24 \text{ g opium}$$

$$0.24 \text{ g opium} \times \frac{10 \text{ g morphine}}{100 \text{ g opium}} \times \frac{1{,}000 \text{ mg}}{1 \text{ g}} = 24 \text{ mg morphine}$$

19. Enough information is available to determine the child's BSA; therefore, this method should be used to calculate the dose because it is more accurate than calculating the dose based on age or weight.

2′4″ = 28″

(BSA from nomogram in Appendix C) = 0.47 m^2

$$\frac{0.47 \text{ m}^2}{1.73 \text{ m}^2} \times 10 \text{ mg} = 2.72 \text{ mg daily}$$

20. $$\frac{100 \text{ mL Elixophyllin}}{180 \text{ mL mixture}} \times \frac{5 \text{ mL mixture}}{1 \text{ dose}} \times \frac{3 \text{ doses}}{1 \text{ day}} = 8.33 \text{ mL Elixophyllin /day}$$

$$\frac{8.33 \text{ mL Elixophyllin}}{1 \text{ day}} \times \frac{80 \text{ mg theophylline}}{15 \text{ mL Elixophyllin}} = 44.44 \text{ mg theophylline/day}$$

21. Amino acids: $\frac{3 \text{ g}}{100 \text{ mL}} \times 1{,}000 \text{ mL} =$

$$30 \text{ g} \times \frac{100 \text{ mL}}{8.5 \text{ g}} = 352.94 \text{ mL}$$

Dextrose: $\frac{15 \text{ g}}{100 \text{ mL}} \times 1{,}000 \text{ mL} =$

$$150 \text{ g} \times \frac{100 \text{ mL}}{50 \text{ g}} = 300 \text{ mL}$$

Sodium chloride:

$$20 \text{ mEq} \times \frac{58.5 \text{ mg}}{1 \text{ mEq}} \times \frac{1 \text{ g}}{1{,}000 \text{ mg}} \times \frac{100 \text{ mL}}{14.6 \text{ g}} = 8.01 \text{ mL}$$

Potassium chloride:

$$25 \text{ mEq} \times \frac{74.5 \text{ mg}}{1 \text{ mEq}} \times \frac{1 \text{ g}}{1{,}000 \text{ mg}} \times \frac{100 \text{ mL}}{14.9 \text{ g}} = 12.5 \text{ mL}$$

Magnesium sulfate:

$$8 \text{ mEq} \times \frac{246 \text{ mg}}{2 \text{ mEq}} \times \frac{1 \text{ g}}{1{,}000 \text{ mg}} \times \frac{100 \text{ mL}}{50 \text{ g}} = 1.97 \text{ mL}$$

Calcium gluconate:

$$10 \text{ mEq} \times \frac{430 \text{ mg}}{2 \text{ mEq}} \times \frac{1 \text{ g}}{1{,}000 \text{ mg}} \times \frac{100 \text{ mL}}{10 \text{ g}} = 21.5 \text{ mL}$$

Potassium phosphate: $15 \text{ mmol} \times \frac{1 \text{ mL}}{3 \text{ mmol}} = 5 \text{ mL}$

Total volume of additives = 701.92 mL

Sterile water for injection: 1,000 mL − 701.92 mL = 298.08 mL

22. $1 \text{ qt solution} \times \frac{2 \text{ pt}}{1 \text{ qt}} \times \frac{473 \text{ mL}}{1 \text{ pt}} \times \frac{1 \text{ g HCl}}{200 \text{ mL solution}} = 4.73 \text{ g HCl}$

$$4.73 \text{ g HCl} \times \frac{100 \text{ g concentrated HCl}}{38 \text{ g HCl}}$$
$$= 12.45 \text{ g concentrated HCl}$$

$$\frac{12.45 \text{ g}}{1.18} = 10.55 \text{ mL}$$

23. Total = 200 parts

Coal tar: $\frac{2 \text{ parts}}{200 \text{ parts}} \times 120 \text{ g} = 1.2 \text{ g}$

Polysorbate 80: $\frac{1 \text{ part}}{200 \text{ parts}} \times 120 \text{ g} = 0.6 \text{ g}$

Zinc oxide paste: $\frac{197 \text{ parts}}{200 \text{ parts}} \times 120 \text{ g} = 118.2 \text{ g}$

24.

Weight (mg)	Absolute Deviation	Deviation Squared
210	$\lvert 210 - 201 \rvert = 9$	81
185	$\lvert 185 - 201 \rvert = 16$	256
200	$\lvert 200 - 201 \rvert = 1$	1
190	$\lvert 190 - 201 \rvert = 11$	121
225	$\lvert 225 - 201 \rvert = 24$	576
205	$\lvert 205 - 201 \rvert = 4$	16
195	$\lvert 195 - 201 \rvert = 6$	36
210	$\lvert 210 - 201 \rvert = 9$	81
200	$\lvert 200 - 201 \rvert = 1$	1
190	$\lvert 190 - 201 \rvert = 11$	121
Totals:		
2,010		1,290

$$\overline{X} = \frac{2{,}010}{10} = 201 \text{ mg}$$

$$\sigma = \sqrt{\frac{1{,}290}{10 - 1}} = \sqrt{143.33} = 11.97 \text{ mg}$$

25. A. $2 \text{ oz} \times \dfrac{28.35 \text{ g}}{1 \text{ oz}} \times \dfrac{1{,}000 \text{ mg}}{1 \text{ g}} \times \dfrac{4{,}400 \text{ units}}{1 \text{ mg}}$

$\times \dfrac{1 \text{ troche}}{400{,}000 \text{ units}} = 623.7 \text{ troches} \approx 623 \text{ troches}$

B. $\dfrac{9}{5} \times 45° + 32° = 113°\text{F}$

References

1. Allen LV, Jr, ed. Ketoprofen 10%, Cyclobenzaprine 1%, and Lidocaine 5% in Poloxamer Lecithin Organogel. Loyd V. Allen, Jr, Editor-in-chief International Journal of Pharmaceutical Compounding 1998;2:154.
2. Prince SJ. Calculations. International Journal of Pharmaceutical Compounding 2002;6:77.
3. Allen LV, Jr, ed. Athletic-Analgesic Rub. Loyd V. Allen, Jr, Editor-in-chief International Journal of Pharmaceutical Compounding 1999;3:130.

Appendices

Appendix A.

Prescription Notation

The use of abbreviated terms and units of measure is common on prescriptions and medication orders. Some terms are derived from the Latin through its historic use in medicine and pharmacy, whereas others have evolved through prescribers' use of writing shortcuts. A list of some common abbreviations is presented in Table A-1. Unfortunately, medication errors can result from the misuse, misinterpretation, and illegible writing of abbreviations, and through the use of ad hoc or made-up abbreviations. The use of a controlled vocabulary, a reduction in the use of abbreviations, care in the writing of decimal points, and the proper use of leading and terminal zeros have been urged to help reduce medication errors.[1–3]

In addition to the use of abbreviations, a prescription also may contain a mixture of Arabic and Roman numerals.

The Roman system of notation is used to express a large range of numbers by the use of eight base letters of the alphabet in a simple "positional" notation to indicate *adding to* or *subtracting from* the succession of letter-values.

The base letters and their values are:

SS or ss = $\frac{1}{2}$	L or l = 50
I or i = 1	C or c = 100
V or v = 5	D or d = 500
X or x = 10	M or m = 1,000

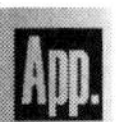

TABLE A-1.
Abbreviations Commonly Used in Prescriptions and Medication Orders

Abbreviation	Meaning
aa. or $\overline{aa}$.	of each
a.c.	before meals
ad	up to; to make
a.d.	right ear
ad lib.	at pleasure, freely
admin.	administer
a.m.	morning
amp.	ampul
aq.	water
a.s.	left ear
ASA	aspirin
ATC	around the clock
a.u.	each ear
b.i.d.	twice a day
BMD	bone mineral density
BM	bowel movement
BP	blood pressure
BS	blood sugar
BSA	body surface area
c. or $\bar{c}$	with
cap.	capsule
cc.	cubic centimeter
CHD	coronary heart disease
CHF	congestive heart failure
comp.	compound
d.	day
dil.	dilute
disc. or DC	discontinue
disp.	dispense
div.	divide
d.t.d.	give of such doses
DW	distilled water

(continued)

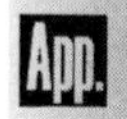

TABLE A-1. *(Continued)*

Abbreviation	Meaning
D5LR	dextrose 5% in lactated Ringer's
D5NS	dextrose 5% in normal saline (0.9% sodium chloride)
D5W	dextrose 5% in water
D10W	dextrose 10% in water
elix.	elixir
e.o.d.	every other day
et	and
ex aq.	in water
f. or fl.	fluid
ft.	make
g	gram
GI	gastrointestinal
gl. aq.	glass of water
GFR	glomerular filtration rate
gtt.	drop
GU	genitourinary
h. or hr.	hour
HA	headache
HBP	high blood pressure
HC	hydrocortisone
HRT	hormone replacement therapy
h.s.	at bedtime
HT or HTN	hypertension
ID	intradermal
IM	intramuscular
inj.	injection
iso.	isotonic
IU	International Units
IV	intravenous
IVP	intravenous push
IVPB	intravenous piggy back
m&n	morning and night
M.	mix

(continued)

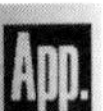

TABLE A-1. *(Continued)*

Abbreviation	Meaning
min.	minute
m^2 or M^2	square meter
mcg	microgram
mEq	milliequivalent
mg	milligram
mg/kg	milligrams (of drug) per kilogram (of body weight)
mg/m^2	milligrams (of drug) per square meter (of body surface area)
mL	milliliter
mL/h	milliliters (of drug administered) per hour (as through intravenous administration)
mOsm or mOsmol	milliosmoles
MI	myocardial ischemia/infarction
MS	morphine sulfate
N&V	nausea and vomiting
NF	National Formulary
NMT	not more than
No.	number
noct.	night
non rep. or N.R.	do not repeat
NPO	nothing by mouth
N.S. or NS	normal saline
1/2NS	half-strength normal saline
NTG	nitroglycerin
o.d.	right eye
o.l.	left eye
o.s.	left eye
o.u.	each eye
o_2	both eyes
oint.	ointment
OJ	orange juice
p.c.	after meals

(continued)

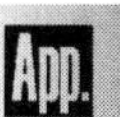

TABLE A-1. *(Continued)*

Abbreviation	Meaning
p.m.	afternoon; evening
p.o.	by mouth
postop	postoperatively
ppm	parts per million
ppb	parts per billion
p.r.n. or prn	when required
pt.	patient
pulv.	powder
q.	every
q.d.	every day
q.h.	every hour
q.i.d.	four times a day
q.o.d.	every other day
q.s. or qs.	a sufficient quantity
q.s. ad	a sufficient quantity to make
rect.	rectal or rectum
rep.	repeat
R.L. or R/L	Ringer's Lactate
℞	prescription symbol (recipe, you take)
s. or $\bar{s}$	without
s.i.d.	once a day
Sig.	write on label
SL	sublingual
SOB	shortness of breath
sol.	solution
s.o.s.	if there is need; as needed
ss. or $\overline{ss}$.	one-half
stat.	immediately
subc or subq or s.c. or SQ	subcutaneously
sup. or supp.	suppository
susp.	suspension
syr.	syrup
tab.	tablet

(continued)

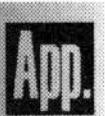

TABLE A-1. *(Continued)*

Abbreviation	Meaning
t.a.t.	until all taken
tbsp.	tablespoonful
t.i.d.	three times a day
t.i.w.	three times a week
top.	topically
TPN	total parenteral nutrition
tsp.	teaspoonful
U or u	unit
u.d. or ut. dict.	as directed
ung.	ointment
URI	upper respiratory infection
USP	United States Pharmacopeia
UTI	urinary tract infection
vol.	volume
w.a.	while awake
wk.	week
fʒi or flʒi	teaspoonful (5 mL)
f℥ss or fl℥ ss	tablespoonful (15 mL)

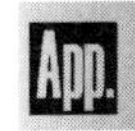

Other quantities are expressed by combining these letters by the general rules:

Two or more letters express a quantity that is the sum of their values if they are successively equal or smaller in value:

Examples:

ii = 2 vi = 6 xii = 12 lxvi = 66 dc = 600
md = 1,500

Two or more letters express a quantity that is the sum of the values remaining after the value of each smaller letter has been subtracted from that of a following greater letter:

Examples:

iv = 4 xiv = 14 xxiv = 24 xl = 40 xc = 90
cdxliv = 444

In pharmacy, Roman numerals generally are used in combination with prescribing abbreviations.

Examples:

M. ft. cap. d.t.d. no. xlviii
Mix and make capsules. Dispense 48 such doses.

gtt. ii o.d. q.d. a.m.
Instill 2 drops into the right eye every day in the morning.

tab. iv stat; tab. ii q6h × 7 d
Take 4 tablets immediately; then take 2 tablets every 6 hours for 7 days.

Tab. i p.r.n. SOB
Take 1 tablet as needed for shortness of breath.

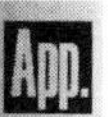

Tab. ii q6h ATC UTI
Take 2 tablets every 6 hours around-the-clock for urinary tract infection.

ʒii q.i.d. p.c. & h.s.
Take 2 teaspoonfuls 4 times per day after meals and at bedtime.

References

1. Davis NM. A controlled vocabulary for reducing medication errors. Hospital Pharmacy 2000;35:227–228.
2. Davis NM. Danger in making 10-fold dosage strengths available. Hospital Pharmacy 1999;34:394.
3. The United States Pharmacopeia. 24th Rev., and National Formulary 19th Ed. Rockville, MD: United States Pharmacopeial Convention, 2000:12.

Appendix B.

Table of Sodium Chloride Equivalents

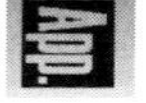

TABLE B.1.
Table of Sodium Chloride Equivalents

Substance	Molecular Weight	Ions	i	Sodium Chloride Equivalent
Antazoline phosphate	363	2	1.8	0.16
Antipyrine	188	1	1.0	0.17
Atropine sulfate $\cdot H_2O$	695	3	2.6	0.12
Benoxinate hydrochloride	345	2	1.8	0.17
Benzalkonium chloride	360	2	1.8	0.16
Benzyl alcohol	108	1	1.0	0.30
Boric acid	61.8	1	1.0	0.52
Chloramphenicol	323	1	1.0	0.10
Chlorobutanol	177	1	1.0	0.24
Chlortetracycline hydrochloride	515	2	1.8	0.11
Cocaine hydrochloride	340	2	1.8	0.16
Cromolyn sodium	512	2	1.8	0.11
Cyclopentolate hydrochloride	328	2	1.8	0.18
Demecarium bromide	717	3	2.6	0.12

(continued)

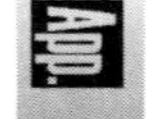

TABLE B-1. *(Continued)*

Substance	Molecular Weight	Ions	i	Sodium Chloride Equivalent
Dextrose (anhydrous)	180	1	1.0	0.18
Dextrose · H_2O	198	1	1.0	0.16
Dipivefrin hydrochloride	388	2	1.8	0.15
Ephedrine hydrochloride	202	2	1.8	0.29
Ephedrine sulfate	429	3	2.6	0.23
Epinephrine bitartrate	333	2	1.8	0.18
Epinephryl borate	209	1	1.0	0.16
Eucatropine hydrochloride	328	2	1.8	0.18
Fluorescein sodium	376	3	2.6	0.31
Glycerin	92	1	1.0	0.34
Homatropine hydrobromide	356	2	1.8	0.17
Hydroxyamphetamine hydrobromide	232	2	1.8	0.25
Idoxuridine	354	1	1.0	0.09
Lidocaine hydrochloride	289	2	1.8	0.22
Mannitol	182	1	1.0	0.18

(continued)

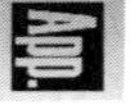

TABLE B-1. *(Continued)*

Substance	Molecular Weight	Ions	i	Sodium Chloride Equivalent
Morphine sulfate · $5H_2O$	759	3	2.6	0.11
Naphazoline hydrochloride	247	2	1.8	0.27
Oxymetazoline hydrochloride	297	2	1.8	0.20
Oxytetracycline hydrochloride	497	2	1.8	0.12
Phenacaine hydrochloride	353	2	1.8	0.20
Phenobarbital sodium	254	2	1.8	0.24
Phenylephrine hydrochloride	204	2	1.8	0.32
Physostigmine salicylate	413	2	1.8	0.16
Physostigmine sulfate	649	3	2.6	0.13
Pilocarpine hydrochloride	245	2	1.8	0.24
Pilocarpine nitrate	271	2	1.8	0.23
Potassium biphosphate	136	2	1.8	0.43
Potassium chloride	74.5	2	1.8	0.76
Potassium iodide	166	2	1.8	0.34
Potassium nitrate	101	2	1.8	0.58

(continued)

TABLE B-1. *(Continued)*

Substance	Molecular Weight	Ions	i	Sodium Chloride Equivalent
Potassium penicillin G	372	2	1.8	0.18
Procaine hydrochloride	273	2	1.8	0.21
Proparacaine hydrochloride	331	2	1.8	0.18
Scopolamine hydrobromide · $3H_2O$	438	2	1.8	0.12
Silver nitrate	170	2	1.8	0.33
Sodium bicarbonate	84	2	1.8	0.65
Sodium borate · $10H_2O$	381	5	4.2	0.42
Sodium carbonate	106	3	2.6	0.80
Sodium carbonate · H_2O	124	3	2.6	0.68
Sodium chloride	58	2	1.8	1.00
Sodium citrate · $2H_2O$	294	4	3.4	0.38
Sodium iodide	150	2	1.8	0.39
Sodium lactate	112	2	1.8	0.52
Sodium phosphate, dibasic, anhydrous	142	3	2.6	0.53
Sodium phosphate, dibasic · $7H_2O$	268	3	2.6	0.29

(continued)

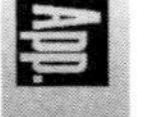

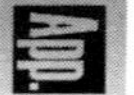

TABLE B-1. *(Continued)*

Substance	Molecular Weight	Ions	i	Sodium Chloride Equivalent
Sodium phosphate, monobasic, anhydrous	120	2	1.8	0.49
Sodium phosphate, monobasic·H_2O	138	2	1.8	0.42
Tetracaine hydrochloride	301	2	1.8	0.18
Tetracycline hydrochloride	481	2	1.8	0.12
Tetrahydrozoline hydrochloride	237	2	1.8	0.25
Timolol maleate	432	2	1.8	0.14
Tobramycin	468	1	1.0	0.07
Tropicamide	284	1	1.0	0.11
Urea	60	1	1.0	0.59
Zinc chloride	136	3	2.6	0.62
Zinc sulfate·$7H_2O$	288	2	1.4	0.15

Appendix C.

Body Surface Area Nomograms

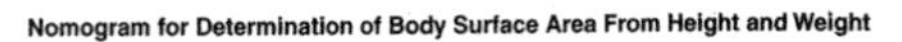

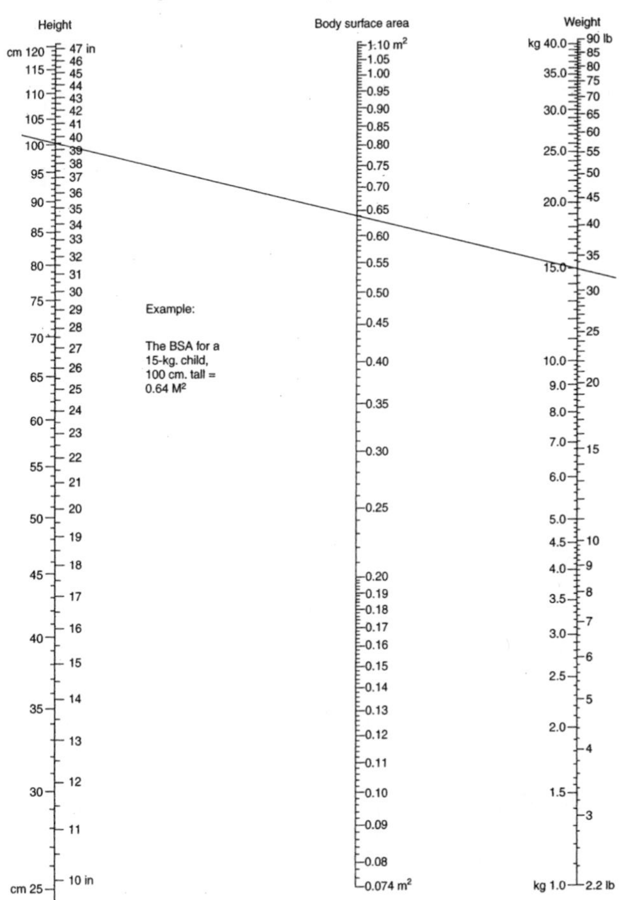

From the formula of Du Bois and Du Bois, *Arch. intern. Med.*, 17, 863 (1916): $S = W^{0.425} \times H^{0.725} \times 71.84$, or $\log S = \log W \times 0.425 + \log H \times 0.725 + 1.8564$ (S = body surface in cm², W = weight in kg, H = height in cm).

FIGURE C-1. Body surface area of children. (Reprinted with permission from Diem K, Lentner C. Documenta Geigy Scientific Tables. 7th Ed. Basel, Switzerland: Geigy Pharmaceuticals, 1970:538.)

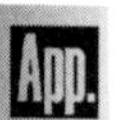

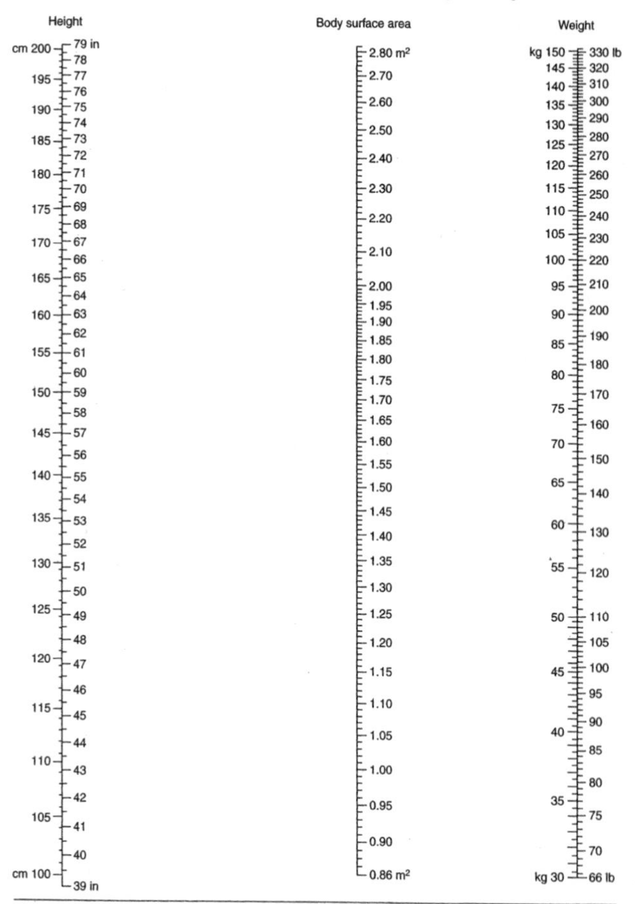

From the formula of Du Bois and Du Bois, *Arch. intern. Med.*, 17, 863 (1916): $S = W^{0.425} \times H^{0.725} \times 71.84$, or $\log S = \log W \times 0.425 + \log H \times 0.725 + 1.8564$ (S = body surface in cm², W = weight in kg, H = height in cm).

FIGURE C-2. Body surface area of adults. (Reprinted with permission from Diem K, Lentner C. Documenta Geigy Scientific Tables. 7th Ed. Basel, Switzerland: Geigy Pharmaceuticals, 1970:537.)

Appendix D.

Table of Atomic Weights

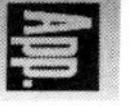

APPENDIX D

Table of Atomic Weights[a]

Name	Symbol	Atomic Number	Weight (Accurate to 4 figures[b])	Approximate Weight
Actinium	Ac	89	227.0	227
Aluminum	Al	13	26.98	27
Americium	Am	95	243.0	243
Antimony	Sb	51	121.8	122
Argon	Ar	18	39.95	40
Arsenic	As	33	74.92	75
Astatine	At	85	209.9	210
Barium	Ba	56	137.3	137
Berkelium	Bk	97	247.0	247
Beryllium	Be	4	9.012	9
Bismuth	Bi	83	208.9	209
Boron	B	5	10.81	11
Bromine	Br	35	79.90	80

(continued)

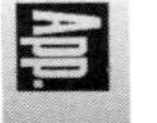

APPENDIX D *(Continued)*

Name	Symbol	Atomic Number	Weight (Accurate to 4 figures[b])	Approximate Weight
Cadmium	Cd	48	112.4	112
Calcium	Ca	20	40.07	40
Californium	Cf	98	251.0	251
Carbon	C	6	12.01	12
Cerium	Ce	58	140.1	140
Cesium	Cs	55	132.9	133
Chlorine	Cl	17	35.45	35
Chromium	Cr	24	51.99	52
Cobalt	Co	27	58.93	59
Copper	Cu	29	63.54	64
Curium	Cm	96	247.0	247
Dysprosium	Dy	66	162.5	163
Einsteinium	Es	99	252.0	252

(continued)

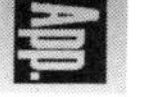

APPENDIX D *(Continued)*

Name	Symbol	Atomic Number	Weight (Accurate to 4 figures[b])	Approximate Weight
Erbium	Er	68	167.2	167
Europium	Eu	63	151.9	152
Fermium	Fm	100	257.0	257
Fluorine	F	9	18.99	19
Francium	Fr	87	223.0	223
Gadolinium	Gd	64	157.2	157
Gallium	Ga	31	69.72	70
Germanium	Ge	32	72.61	73
Gold	Au	79	196.9	197
Hafnium	Hf	72	178.4	179
Helium	He	2	4.003	4
Holmium	Ho	67	164.9	165
Hydrogen	H	1	1.008	1

(continued)

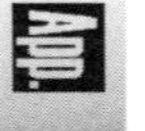

APPENDIX D *(Continued)*

Name	Symbol	Atomic Number	Weight (Accurate to 4 figures[b])	Approximate Weight
Indium	In	49	114.8	115
Iodine	I	53	126.9	127
Iridium	Ir	77	192.2	192
Iron	Fe	26	55.85	56
Krypton	Kr	36	83.80	84
Lanthanum	La	57	138.9	139
Lawrencium	Lr	103	262.1	262
Lead	Pb	82	207.2	207
Lithium	Li	3	6.941	7
Lutetium	Lu	71	174.9	175
Magnesium	Mg	12	24.31	24
Manganese	Mn	25	54.94	55
Mendelevium	Md	101	258.1	258

(continued)

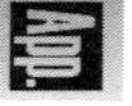

APPENDIX D *(Continued)*

Name	Symbol	Atomic Number	Weight (Accurate to 4 figures[b])	Approximate Weight
Mercury	Hg	80	200.6	201
Molybdenum	Mo	42	95.94	96
Neodymium	Nd	60	144.2	144
Neon	Ne	10	20.18	20
Neptunium	Np	93	237.0	237
Nickel	Ni	28	58.69	59
Niobium	Nb	41	92.91	93
Nitrogen	N	7	14.01	14
Nobelium	No	102	259.1	259
Osmium	Os	76	190.2	190
Oxygen	O	8	16.00	16
Palladium	Pd	46	106.4	106
Phosphorus	P	15	30.97	31

(continued)

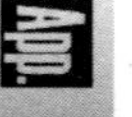

APPENDIX D *(Continued)*

Name	Symbol	Atomic Number	Weight (Accurate to 4 figures[b])	Approximate Weight
Platinum	Pt	78	195.1	195
Plutonium	Pu	94	244.1	244
Polonium	Po	84	208.9	209
Potassium	K	19	39.10	39
Praseodymium	Pr	59	140.9	141
Promethium	Pm	61	144.9	145
Protactinium	Pa	91	231.0	231
Radium	Ra	88	226.0	226
Radon	Rn	86	222.0	222
Rhenium	Re	75	186.2	186
Rhodium	Rh	45	102.9	103
Rubidium	Rb	37	85.47	85
Ruthenium	Ru	44	101.1	101

(continued)

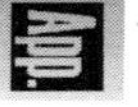

APPENDIX D *(Continued)*

Name	Symbol	Atomic Number	Weight (Accurate to 4 figures[b])	Approximate Weight
Samarium	Sm	62	150.4	150
Scandium	Sc	21	44.96	45
Selenium	Se	34	78.96	79
Silicon	Si	14	28.09	28
Silver	Ag	47	107.9	108
Sodium	Na	11	22.99	23
Strontium	Sr	38	87.62	88
Sulfur	S	16	32.07	32
Tantalum	Ta	73	180.9	181
Technetium	Tc	43	97.91	98
Tellurium	Te	52	127.6	128
Terbium	Tb	65	158.9	159
Thallium	Tl	81	204.4	204
Thorium	Th	90	232.0	232

(continued)

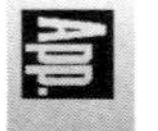

APPENDIX D *(Continued)*

Name	Symbol	Atomic Number	Weight (Accurate to 4 figures[b])	Approximate Weight
Thulium	Tm	69	168.9	169
Tin	Sn	50	118.7	119
Titanium	Ti	22	47.88	48
Tungsten	W	74	183.9	184
Unnilhexium	Unh	106	263.2	263
Unnilpentium	Unp	105	262.1	262
Unnilquadium	Unq	104	261.1	261
Unnilseptium	Uns	107	262.1	262
Uranium	U	92	238.0	238
Vanadium	V	23	50.94	51
Xenon	Xe	54	131.3	131
Ytterbium	Yb	70	173.0	173
Yttrium	Y	39	88.91	89

(continued)

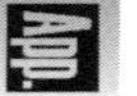

APPENDIX D *(Continued)*

Name	Symbol	Atomic Number	Weight (Accurate to 4 figures[b])	Approximate Weight
Zinc	Zn	30	65.39	65
Zirconium	Zr	40	91.22	91

[a] Derived from the table recommended in 1981 by the Commission on Atomic Weights of the International Union of Pure and Applied Chemistry. All atomic weight values are based on the atomic mass of $^{12}C = 12$.

[b] When rounded off to 4-figure accuracy, these weights are practically identical to the similarly rounded-off weights in the older table based on oxygen = 16.0000.

Index

Page numbers set in *italics* denote figures; those followed by a t denote tables.